PEAK PERFORMANCE ON PLANTS

—

The Essential Guide to Vegan Nutrition for Everyone from Competitive Athletes to Couch Potatoes

Alex Wood
&
Aisha Summers

For the animals
A. W.

For Sofia & Rafi
A. S.

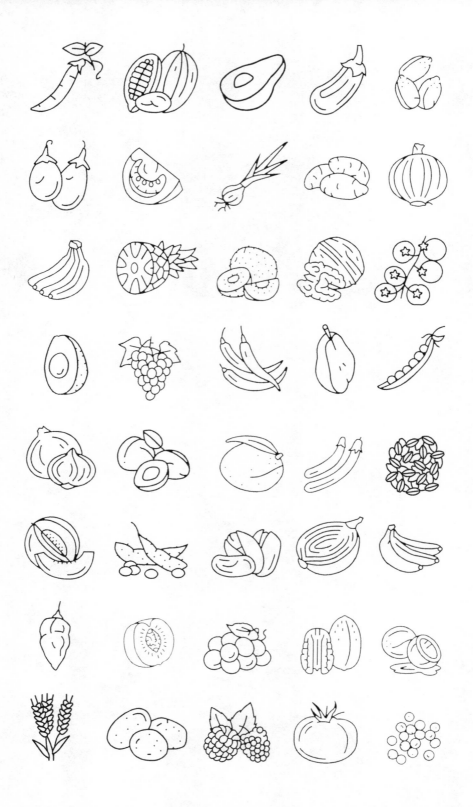

CONTENTS

INTRODUCTION

When I was a kid in middle school, I don't think I was all that cool. I was good at sports, I played football and basketball. I wasn't the best on the team, but I wasn't the worst either. I kept my head down, I did my schoolwork. I always remember those kids who knew what the hottest thing was going to be before everybody else did. They would have seen the new blockbuster before it was released in the movie theatres, or they'd have been listening to the band that went mainstream long before the rest of us had even heard their name. If you were born in the 1980s or before, I'm sure you know the kind of person I'm talking about. This was all before the age of social media, a time when people still regularly went to the movie theater and bought music by the album.

Anyway, the irony is that now I've become that kind of person – but I wasn't into a band before everyone else. I was into veganism. I've been vegan for decades, since long before it was as widespread as it is now. And long before it was as easy as it is now! I've seen it change from the super unfashionable fringe to becoming a lifestyle that influencers are using to promote their own personal brand.

I stopped using animal products in college. I was on the track team at the time and my coach told me in no uncertain terms that if I didn't start eating meat, I'd be dropped from the team. I was surprised because at the time my 400m was steadily improving. It might have been team politics or the people I was hanging out with off the track, but I'm pretty sure that kind of call would never be made today. I quit the team on principle. A personal experience had opened my eyes to what we humans were doing to the other species on the planet, and that seemed way more important than anything else. It still does. It changed my life completely.

But I didn't write this book to tell you my life story. You've got your own story, and it may or may not involve veganism. Most likely it involves something adjacent, which is why you're reading this book.

Maybe you're on the edges, you still eat meat and dairy, but you want to make a move towards a more plant-based diet. Maybe you're worried that this kind of change will result in a loss of power or performance and your head is filled by the voices of the bros at the gym who swear by the carnivore diet. Or maybe you've been eating plant-based for a while now, and that initial rush of energy that you felt at the start has begun to dwindle. Maybe you're hitting the wall more often than you want to and your training isn't at the sweet spot that you know it can be. Or maybe, even, you've been in it for the long haul like me. What if you've been a vegan for years and you know how to cook and you know what you like to eat, but what if you could make a few changes that would drastically improve your energy levels? What if you could lift yourself out of the plateau you've found yourself drifting along?

Your story is what's important here. How can you use the things that you eat to do what you do at your best?

Humans are a complex piece of organic machinery that runs on food. To work at our best, we need the right kind of food. We are omnivores, we can eat everything, but if you've made the change to cutting out animal products from your diet – or are thinking of making it – then you need to know how to optimize your nutrition to get the best results.

Confused about where to begin?

This book is here to help. It's packed full of information about plant-based nutrition – why it matters, and how it can benefit your body. Whether you want to lose weight, boost energy levels, or reduce your risk of chronic disease, this book will show you why a plant-based diet is important.

There's a lot of noise about plant-based diets in the media, and it's hard to know who to listen to. Often those who are shouting the loudest seem the most authoritative, but they might not be giving you the complete picture. This book aims to do exactly that, to give you the facts, so you can make up your mind about what's best for you.

Before we begin though – and at the risk of sounding like I only want to talk about myself – I do need to tell you a little bit more about myself. Actually, it's not just about me, it's about us. I'm not writing this book on my own. It's a team effort, and I'm only one half of the team.

My name is Alex Wood, and I've been vegan for more than two decades. Without trying to sound full of it, I'm still in the best shape of my life. I've competed in Iron Man and body building competitions, and continue to run a successful personal training business, all while eating an exclusively plant-based diet. I've tried it all. I've coached countless clients into improving their personal bests and changing the way they eat to include more conscious choices. It would be very easy for me to sing the praises of a vegan diet and say that by going plant-based you can do no wrong. That's what I want to do! As far as I'm concerned, the less suffering that animals face the better!

However, I understand it's not as simple as that. Everyone has different needs and requirements, and overselling vegan hype sometimes generates the opposite reaction from the effect you want. If you only tell one side of the story, people can see right through it. To give you a more balanced view, I'm writing this book with Aisha Summers, a nutritionist and popular science writer. We're going to look at what current research says about plant-based diets, in particular to how they relate to performance. For full disclosure, Aisha isn't vegan – she eats a high percentage of plant-based foods, but also consumes some animal products. First and foremost, she tries to follow scientific principles, to look for sound evidence to back up claims made about health and nutrition. This is what she is going to provide in this book: an unbiased approach to the complex and outspoken field of vegan nutrition.

So, although this book has been written by the two of us, it's mainly going to come from one voice to be less confusing. There will be plenty of references to all the research – it's all listed in the back of the book, so you can dig deeper into the studies if you are interested. I may make my own personal preferences known but won't let that get in your way. I want you to make the most informed decision you can for your health. If my opinion differs from what the science says, I'll make it clear.

You will find practical advice on everything from food choices and meal planning to timing and supplementation, we'll break down the science behind plant-based nutrition into simple terms that you can easily understand.

We'll start by looking at what plant-based nutrition is and dispel some of the myths that surround it. You might be surprised to learn that a plant-based diet isn't necessarily vegetarian or vegan - it's simply a way of eating that focuses on plants, rather than animal products. This may already be very obvious to you.

We'll then explore the science behind plant-based nutrition and discover how it can help improve your health in several ways. We'll look at how plant-based nutrition can reduce your risk of chronic diseases such as heart disease, diabetes, and cancer. We'll also look more generally at the connection between nutrition and performance.

Then we'll take a look at all the main food groups and how they fit into your diet, what to eat when you need more energy or protein, and the best strategies for getting those nutrients from plants instead of animal products. Some of the most important information in this book is about what – if anything – is missing from a plant-based diet, and whether any of the nutrients you need are harder to obtain from plants alone.

We'll also talk about gut health, timing your meals for maximum results, and other important factors that can help you get the most out of your plant-based lifestyle. Whether you're new to plant-based eating or are looking for ways to optimize your nutrition, this book will provide a comprehensive guide to keeping your body at its best – *on plants!*

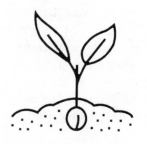

CHAPTER 1

WHAT DO YOU MEAN "PLANT-BASED"?

If it came from a plant, eat it; if it was made in a plant, don't.

Michael Pollan

Michael Pollan is a well-known food writer and advocate for plant-based diets. His views reflect his concern for both personal health and ecological sustainability, views which have now become widespread. The interaction between these two things is what we are going to cover in this chapter.

We are going start things off by defining basic terminology used when it comes to eating plant based. We'll also cover the reasons why people start eating a plant-based diet, from environmental considerations to ethics and health. We'll introduce the idea of a whole food diet, and how it can be different from a plant-based one, and how the energy density and nutrient density of foods are connected. There's a lot to cover, so let's get going!

What is a plant-based diet?

This is obvious, but let's go over it anyway. At its most basic, plant-based nutrition refers to diets that are centered on foods derived from plants, such as fruits, vegetables, legumes, grains, nuts, and seeds. This type of diet can be either vegetarian, vegan or neither – it simply focuses on plant-based foods rather than animal products.

WHY CHOOSE A PLANT-BASED DIET?

There are many reasons, and everyone has their own. Some, like me, do it for ethical reasons, as they believe it is wrong to cause any kind of harm or suffering to animals (or to humans for that matter). Others do it for environmental reasons, as the industrialization of animal agriculture has become a major contributor to greenhouse gas emissions and other forms of pollution. A growing number have started to do it for health reasons, as a plant-based diet has been shown to reduce the risk of various chronic diseases. And finally, some do it for religious reasons, as some religions require or encourage followers to consume a plant-based diet – this is ultimately an ethical reason.

While going plant-based can have many benefits, it is important to note that it is not a magic solution to all of your or the world's problems. Animal agriculture is just one of many industries that contribute to environmental degradation, and a plant-based diet is not necessarily healthy if it is not well-planned. If you are interested in reducing your impact on animals and the environment, a plant-based diet is a good place to start, but like everything of value, needs your continued input and attention to make sure it is working at its best.

THE TEMPERATURE'S RISING

It is no secret that the global vegan population is on the rise. In 2021, it was estimated that there were 79 million vegans around the world,[1] and this number is only increasing. The vegan food market is also growing rapidly, reaching a value of over $16 billion in 2021.[2] One of the biggest reasons behind this trend is that for many people, the decision to go vegan is motivated by environmental concerns.

Animal products are responsible for a significant amount of greenhouse gas emissions, approximately 57% of total global emissions for food come from animal agriculture, according to some estimates.[3] Beef is by far the biggest source of emissions, followed by lamb, pork, and dairy. But beyond recognizing that the farming of animals produces a huge amount of greenhouse gasses (not just from farming processes, but also from the cattle themselves in the form of methane burps), it is surprisingly hard to evaluate the effect of cutting out animal products on greenhouse gas emissions. One modelling study from 2012 showed that choosing the vegan option would only reduce the emission of greenhouse gases by 3% per person.[4] Another study from 2018 estimated a much higher 20-30%.[5]

The picture is further complicated by considering what you might eat on a vegan diet. If you eat a lot of out of season fruit, or water hungry Californian almonds or avocados, for instance, you will drive up the impact your diet has on the environment. If you live in a cold country and want to eat soft fruit in the winter that needs to be air freighted in to stay fresh, then the carbon footprint of your diet expands dramatically. In extreme cases, this can mean that your diet will have a more detrimental impact on the environment than eating a little bit of meat from responsible sources.

There's also the issue of crops like soy or wheat, which are often grown in vast pesticide and insecticide-soaked monocultures. Often those who want to defend animal farming point out that these crops cause a large amount of deforestation. This leads to soil degradation, destroys habitats, and contributes to a decrease in biodiversity. However, much of the soy and wheat that is grown ends up being used for animal feed, and some estimates show that if everyone went vegan, we could produce enough food to feed everyone with 75% less space. Producing crops to feed animals and then eating the animals is incredibly energy inefficient. It takes about 6kg of plant protein to produce 1kg of animal protein.[6] Over 80% of farmland is used for livestock, but it produces just 18% of food calories. The numbers are crazy.

However, the story isn't always completely clear cut. Animals like cows and sheep, which are ruminants, can eat a lot of the plant matter that is indigestible to humans, so it is not as simple as producing food that is directly fed to animals. They add efficiency into the food chain by eating what would otherwise be waste. Likewise, sometimes the land that they feed on is marginal and impossible to farm for crops. The other side of the story has some good points.

So, how much impact a plant-based diet has on the environment is debatable, but one big study published in Science in 2018 led the head researcher to conclude: "A vegan diet is probably the single biggest way to reduce your impact on planet Earth, not just greenhouse gases, but global acidification, eutrophication, land use and water use. It is far bigger than cutting down on your flights or buying an electric car."[7]

PRO-LIFE

Many vegans are motivated by concerns for animal welfare. They believe that just because humans are stronger and intellectually more capable, that does not give us the right to oppress and abuse other species. I fall into this category. Vegans like me believe we have a responsibility to care for other animals, just like we should care for other humans. If a conscious being is capable of suffering, we shouldn't cause it suffering through our own selfish actions.

However, you might side with René Descartes, the 17th Century French philosopher and mathematician, who argued that animals aren't conscious, and therefore it's absolutely fine to cause them physical or emotional pain and kill them. If you've ever spent any time with an animal, that probably seems like a ridiculous conclusion to come to. Scientific consensus agrees with you. In 2012, through "The Cambridge Declaration on Consciousness," a group of neuroscientists agreed that animals have the "neurobiological substrates of conscious experience" and are capable of experiencing affective states. Affective states are not just quick responses to stimuli, but mood states, like anxiety or depression.[8]

We've come to understand the strength of the mother-child bond, and how powerful hormonal systems establish it. We understand that similar systems exist in both humans and animals, yet we consistently create the bond and then break it in order to put milk in our coffee. The dairy industry runs on taking babies away from their mothers and then impregnating the mothers so that they continue to produce milk. This process is repeated over and over again until the cow is no longer capable of fulfilling this function and turned into ground beef. Ethical vegans believe this causes incredible distress to the animals involved and have decided not to take part in the process by refusing to buy and consume the products that the process creates.

Again, the numbers are crazy here. One source estimates that 271 land animals are killed every second in the United States alone.[9] In 2019, 72 billion chickens were slaughtered worldwide for food (more than 2,000 a second). In the US, more than a quarter of the meat produced isn't even eaten, it's just thrown away.[10]

PRO-HEALTH

Some vegans are motivated by health concerns, and they avoid all animal products to improve their health or to prevent disease. Increasing volumes of research are finding links between consuming animal products and chronic disease. This is the subject of a chapter in itself, Chapter 3, so we will wait until then to go over it in detail.

WHAT'S THE DIFFERENCE BETWEEN VEGAN AND PLANT-BASED?

Although the terms "vegan" and "plant-based" are often used interchangeably, there is an obvious difference between the two. A vegan diet excludes all animal products, including meat, dairy, eggs, and honey. A plant-based diet is mostly or entirely based on plants. This includes fruits, vegetables, grains, legumes, nuts, and seeds, but it does not exclude anything. So, all vegans are plant-based, but not all plant-based eaters are vegan. For example, someone who follows a plant-based diet but occasionally eats fish would not be considered vegan.

Some will also argue that the term "vegan" inherently carries an ethical dimension, and that you can only call yourself a vegan if you're in it for the animals. To me it depends how militant you want to be, but veganism is really more than a diet. I'm happy for someone to call themselves vegan, even if they're only doing it for health reasons, as long as they don't use animal products of any sort. That means no leather shoes or woolen sweaters as well. Vegans are against the commodification of animals in any form.

OTHER TERMS FOR PLANT-BASED EATERS

You've probably come across all of these before. Many try one of the first two before making the dive into full veganism.

Lacto-ovo vegetarian: Lacto-ovo vegetarian diets are among the most traditional vegetarian diets. You avoid meat and fish in this variation, but you consume eggs and dairy products.

Pescatarian: In a pescatarian diet, fish (from the Italian pesce) is included. Pescatarian diets often also include dairy products and eggs depending on an individual's preferences. One perceived benefit of the pescatarian diet is that you get a healthy dose of omega-3 fatty acids from eating fatty fish, something which we will see can be difficult to obtain on particular kinds of purely plant-based diets.[11] However, eating fish comes with its own set of potential health problems, and some types of fishing can be very damaging to the environment.

Flexitarian: Most plant-based eaters nowadays have become flexitarian – especially if the reason for cutting out meat isn't ethical. The diet is more versatile than a strictly vegetarian or vegan one. Plant-based foods are emphasized, but animal products in small quantities are allowed.

Raw Vegan: Those who follow a raw vegan diet do not consume cooked foods at all. Raw vegans only eat raw plants or foods that have been heated between temperatures of 104-118° F (40-48° C). They claim that the nutritional value of raw and minimally heated foods is higher than that of cooked foods. In particular, enzymes, which are heat sensitive, will still be present in the food and the water-soluble vitamins won't be lost. This type of diet is subject to some scrutiny because many vegetables such as tomatoes and asparagus are made more nutritionally valuable when they are cooked before consumption, and there have been no studies showing that a lack of food enzymes in the food itself causes any problems. Our bodies produce all the enzymes we need to break down the food we eat.

Finally, there is also the term "veggan," used to describe someone who follows a vegan diet but occasionally eats eggs. There is the term "beegan", which is used to describe someone who follows a plant-based diet but occasionally eats honey. And there are "freegans" who are vegans that scavenge for food and will sometimes eat meat if it would otherwise have gone to waste. These are all essentially forms of flexitarianism and to be honest, I've not yet met someone who calls themselves veggan or beegan!

THE WHOLE FOOD DIET

Although many people become vegan for health reasons, just because a diet is vegan definitely doesn't mean that it is healthy.

I've met plenty of people who have assumed that my vegan diet is super healthy because they have confused it with a whole food diet. A whole food diet is one where you avoid processed foods as much as possible. Whole foods are the closest you can get to their unrefined natural form. Although this is a vague and ill-defined term, it makes a certain amount of intuitive sense. Often the advice given is not to eat anything that comes prepackaged, or anything that contains more than five ingredients, or anything that you grandmother wouldn't recognize as food.

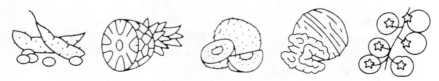

On a whole food diet, you can eat:

- Whole grains
- Milk and some dairy products
- Vegetables and fruits
- Eggs
- Meat, poultry, and seafood
- Nuts and seeds
- Legumes and beans

What you can't eat:

- Processed foods
- Foods and drinks with added sugars
- Packaged ready to eat foods
- Refined grains
- Vegetable oils

So, to put it into practical food terms, think of having a baked potato, rather than a big bag of potato chips or have a bowl of oatmeal and raspberries, rather than a dried fruit breakfast bar.

In a whole food diet, there is some ambiguity when it comes to meat. Even though it definitely counts as a whole food, most of the meat and poultry sold in the market contains antibiotics and hormones, which is problematic. The same holds with dairy. Even if milk comes from an organic source, it is processed by being pasteurized. If you were being strict with the diet, then organic animal products could be chosen instead, and raw milk drunk, or meat and dairy avoided entirely. Even if you are not eating animal products, the diet can be open to interpretation. For instance, some prefer to soak and prepare dry beans at home instead of using canned "processed" beans. If you're being very strict with the diet, you might not use anything that has been pre-processed.

Neither "whole food" or "processed" are precisely defined terms, and if you're planning to follow a whole food diet, you need to come up with an interpretation that you're satisfied with. How strict you want to be with the diet is up to you and boils down to what level of processing you're willing to accept. And as you can see, a whole food diet doesn't necessarily have to be 100% plant-based unless you want it to be. The only plant-based diet that is unequivocally whole food is a raw vegan diet.

There are many benefits to eating a whole food diet. One of the most important is that it can help you to avoid the unhealthy additives and chemicals that are often found in processed foods. It also can help you to get more nutrients and fiber in your diet, less added sugars and fats, and therefore can help you to maintain a healthy weight.

If you're interested in following a whole food diet, especially a plant-based one, the best thing you can do is to cook at home using fresh, unprocessed ingredients. This will give you more control over what you eat and allow you to avoid processed foods altogether. Nowadays, if you go out to eat vegan food, it's hard to get anything which hasn't been highly processed. In fact, this has been the greatest problem with the runaway expansion of the vegan market: the rise of vegan junk food.

THE PROBLEM WITH PROCESSED FOOD

Let me first clarify that not all forms of processing are unhealthy. For example, when you cook a tomato, you are technically processing it. However, we know that cooking increases the availability of certain nutrients in tomatoes such as lycopene and carotenoids both of which are antioxidants that play a protective role for the cells in our body. There is also plenty of research showing that fermented foods are beneficial for gut and brain health.[12] Sprouting grains enhances their amino acid profile and sugar composition, as well as their digestibility. These are all foods that have been lightly processed and have a greater nutrient density than they might have had before.

The foods that we really want to avoid are those that have been heavily processed or the ones that have been made with ultra-processed ingredients. In a heavily processed food, components are usually extracted from whole foods – the most commonly consumed ones are oil and sugar, but often protein is extracted from plants or dairy, and even MSG, some food dyes and stabilizers also come from natural sources. Some components are produced from components not normally considered food – for instance artificial food dyes like Red 40, Yellow 5 and Yellow 6 which are made from petroleum. Different foods are processed for different reasons, but mostly it is for convenience, shelf life, or to make them more palatable. This can obviously be detrimental to your health, since it means adding excessive sugar, salt, unhealthy fats, chemical and artificial ingredients. All of this has been shown to have negative health outcomes, from causing weight gain to an increased risk of high blood pressure, type 2 diabetes, depression, irritable bowel syndrome and overall incidence of cancer.[13]

They are also bad for your brain and your heart. The outcome of a large study involving over a hundred thousand participants showed that eating ultra-processed foods increased the likelihood of coronary heart disease and cerebrovascular disease.[14] This conclusion was reached after researchers accounted for levels of sugar, sodium, fiber, and saturated fat consumption in the diets. Furthermore, in another large study, the findings showed that eating more than four servings of processed food daily was associated with a higher risk of death from all causes. There was an 18% increase in mortality risk for each additional serving.[15]

The goal of a whole food diet is to eliminate all kinds of processed foods and rather focus on foods that are dense in nutrients. This brings us to an interesting theory about how to decide what the healthiest choice of food is, based on its nutrient-density and calorie content.

DR FUHRMAN'S HEALTH EQUATION

Dr Joel Fuhrman is a Board-certified family physician, nutritional researcher, and bestselling author who specializes in preventative medicine. In his book *Eat to Live*, Dr. Fuhrman introduces his 'principles of health' equation as a way of simplifying food choices and maximizing nutrition. I have found this to be such a powerful way of looking at food that I often recommend it to my clients who are just starting out and are struggling with food choices because they have long been dependent on processed foods.

The equation is as follows: "Health" = nutrients / calories

I've put "health" in inverted commas, because it works best if thought of in broad terms. We're not looking at specific measurable outcomes, like dyslipidemia or insulin sensitivity, or even broader ideas like weight loss or muscle gain, but overall glowing, feeling-on-top-of-the-world, not-about-to-die-anytime-soon health. And the nutrients we're talking about are not the ones associated with calories, like carbohydrates, proteins, and fats, but the micronutrients – the vitamins and minerals. So, in simple terms, the healthiest choice is the food which contains the highest proportion of these micronutrients for the lowest number of calories. If you're getting a huge dose of phytochemicals and antioxidants whilst simultaneously not having an oversupply of calories, your health will benefit. Simple, right?

NUTRIENT DENSITY - WHAT DOES IT MEAN? WHY DOES IT MATTER?

Fuhrman's idea isn't unique, he's just created a good way of transmitting the information. A health equation is catchy and memorable. Others have also tried to determine the nutrient density of various foods. In most methods, a score is assigned to the food based on the average of percent daily values for a selection of different nutrients that you'd find in 100 grams of the food.[16]

The United States Centre for Disease Control and Prevention (CDC) took this up and came up with its own branding, defining what it called "Powerhouse fruits and vegetables."[17] At the top of the list with the highest nutrient density scores were cruciferous and leafy green vegetables, like watercress, chard, and spinach. At the bottom were sweet potato and grapefruit. Ironically, neither avocados nor blueberries – fruits that are often at the top of internet "superfood" lists – made it onto the CDC's list. Garlic and onions didn't satisfy the criteria either, and they're some of the foods that Dr Fuhrman suggests you should eat every day because of their tremendous nutritional benefit.

It goes to show that a lot of nutritional "information" can end up being a form of branding that might well have an agenda behind it. The label "superfood" definitely is, and "Powerhouse fruits and vegetables" too. Fuhrman's health equation is catchy but ill-defined. The idea of "health" isn't quantified in any way, and like all good branding, it is ultimately used to sell his products and services.

However, that doesn't stop it all being useful to help you think about food choices. Generally, a whole food diet is going to have a higher nutrient density. Nutrient density is also negatively correlated with energy density – energy-dense foods tend to be nutrient-poor.

NUTRIENT DENSITY VS ENERGY DENSITY

A food's energy density is simply determined by the number of calories it contains per 100 grams, which has no connection to its nutritional value. Foods with a high energy density have more calories per gram than foods with a low energy density. Foods and beverages vary in energy density depending on their water, carbohydrate, protein, and fat content. Low-energy foods, such as certain fruits and vegetables, tend to have a higher water and fiber content.

A large meta-analysis of over 3,000 obese adults examining multiple experimental and observational studies showed that consuming low-energy-density foods significantly affected body weight.[18] To put it simply, individuals who consumed more nutritionally dense, low-calorie foods like vegetables and fruit, whole grains, and legumes were less likely to be overweight than people who consumed calorie-dense, lower-nutrient foods such as fast food. That seems intuitively obvious, but it is backed up by some research. And remember, just because a food is plant-based, it doesn't mean it has a high nutrient or low energy density.

Although it may be tempting to equate nutrient-dense foods with low-calorie foods, or energy-dense foods with little nutrients, it isn't always the case. It's true that the most nutrient-dense foods tend to have a low energy density, however there are foods which are nutritious and have a high energy content. Nuts, seeds and avocados are the obvious ones in the plant-based world. If you eat animal products, then organ meats are particularly high in nutrients, even though they contain quite a lot of calories too. Likewise, some foods are low in calories, like celery, cucumber and iceberg lettuce, and also have a fairly low nutrient density.

Getting fixated on the density of nutrients or energy in your food won't necessarily mean you have the best diet. The best diet is the one that you can stick to. Rather than having one fixed set of rules, it is better to be flexible, as your overall dietary goals can be reached by combining foods of varying nutritional and energy content. Ideally, healthy diets meet nutritional needs by including whole foods that are high in nutrients (for instance dark leafy greens), but they can also include foods that aren't so healthy if they're consumed occasionally and in moderation (such as fruit juices). If you consume more highly processed foods, it's important to make sure they make up only a small percentage of the diet. Moderation and variety are key factors in ensuring you reach the optimum nutrient-to-energy ratio and that you actually stick to your eating plan!

THE PROBLEM WITH 'CLEAN EATING'

I hear it less often than I used to, but there are still plenty of trainers and social media influencers around who claim that their motto is, "Eat clean, train dirty." I don't really like either side of that equation. It's an outdated idea that you've got to be destroyed on the floor of the gym to have had a successful workout, just like it's unnecessary to think of your food as "clean."

In recent years, there has been a growing trend of people trying to eat more "clean" foods. Clean eating is often marketed as a way to lose weight, boost energy levels, and improve overall health. But what does it really mean? That's the first problem: the term is imprecise and can mean different things to different people. For some people, clean eating simply means eating more whole foods and avoiding processed ones. For others, it might mean following a very specific diet such as the Paleo diet or being a raw vegan. For others it means cutting out almost everything that could be considered detrimental to your health. Considering the uncertainties and contradictions in the realm of nutrition science, this might result in cutting out a lot.

This can mean that it's often seen as an all-or-nothing approach to food. You're either eating "clean" or you're not. You might feel guilty if you slip up and eat something that isn't considered "clean." It perpetuates the idea that some foods are "good", and some foods are "bad." This creates a judgmental attitude towards food and can make you feel distressed or anxious for eating what you have arbitrarily labelled as the wrong thing.

It can also lead to an unhealthy obsession with food and an unrealistic view of what is possible to achieve in terms of nutrition. This can lead to disordered eating behaviors such as restrictive dieting and orthorexia. Orthorexia is an unhealthy obsession with eating healthy food, and people who suffer from it become so obsessed that it starts to seriously interfere with their daily lives.[19]

And of course, another problem with clean eating is that it's often used as a way to sell products. The wellness industry has latched onto the trend and is using it to sell everything from supplements to cookbooks. While there is nothing wrong with selling products that can help people eat more healthily and improve their lives, the problem is that these products are often unnecessary, overpriced, and inadequately supported by science.

If you're interested in having a healthier diet, there's nothing wrong with wanting to eat more of what you perceive to be a better choice of food, but it's important to recognize that labelling what you're eating as "clean" might cause you more problems than it solves. Use less judgmental terminology, like whole foods, or better yet, something objective that can be quantified, like nutrient density. Be mindful of the way that clean eating is marketed today. Make sure that you're making choices that are best for your overall health, not just following the latest food trend.

MY VEGAN JOURNEY

I've experimented with various different styles of veganism throughout the twenty-five years I've been eating a wholly plant-based diet. Some were better than others. I couldn't stick with being raw, it just didn't work for me. I lasted less than two weeks. I felt hungry all the time and often a little irritable, and I felt like I was constantly eating in order to get enough calories in. I also lost more weight than I wanted to – I found it was almost impossible to keep the muscle on.

I've had periods of eating mainly whole foods and trying to cut out processed foods; I've had times when I've relied on extracted proteins from pea, soya, and hemp to make protein shakes; and I've even had periods of indulging in my fair share of vegan junk food. I've definitely felt great on a whole food diet but have found the macro-nutrition side more challenging. The level of performance I've expected from my body has been impacted by my diet. A whole food plant-based diet was great when I was training for triathlons and set me up well for the Ironman but didn't work out well for bodybuilding or Olympic lifting at all. And that's for me. You might be a different matter.

I've never tried to reintroduce animal products back into my diet although I know that has been the right call for some of my clients. I've found that my diet has needed to change depending on what I've been doing at the time. What I've eaten has had to match the kind of performance that's needed from my body and mind, and this is going to be the subject of the next chapter.

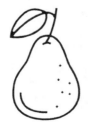

CHAPTER 2

WHAT DO YOU WANT TO DO?

If you fail to prepare, you're prepared to fail.

Mark Spitz

You aren't what you eat, but what you eat will determine what you can do. The term "performance" is often used for athletes, and this is my area of expertise. I've spent years coaching athletes to improve physical fitness, to reach performance goals, and get the most out of their body. I've worked with everyone from professional sportspeople and weekend warriors to new parents trying to get back into shape and overworked executives trying to fight middle-age spread. And I've worked with people who have been trying hard to rebuild their health after some very serious complications and problems.

When looking at the effect of diet on performance, we need to broaden our scope. Achieving peak performance isn't solely the domain of traditional athleticism. There are many activities which require high performance but aren't considered athletic. A notable example is chess, notable because popular culture often portrays chess as the least athletic endeavor possible.

According to Robert Sapolsky, chess grandmasters can burn up to 6,000 calories daily while competing in tournaments. Sapolsky studies stress in primates and found that grandmasters are experiencing stress in a similar way to elite athletes: chess competitions triple respiratory rates, elevate blood pressure, and cause muscle contractions to increase. Sapolsky says, "Grand-masters sustain elevated blood pressure for hours in the range found in competitive marathon runners."[1]

Ultimately performance is also relative. Maybe you're not a traditional "athlete" or a chess grandmaster. Maybe you're like most of us who want to do the best we can with what we've got right now.

PERFORMANCE

We can think of performance simply as the ability of the body to physically perform, whether that means running a marathon or being able to walk up a flight of stairs without getting winded or even just being able to sit comfortably and concentrate.

Many different factors can impact someone's performance, especially nutrition. What you eat will directly affect your physical performance, and often it can feel immediate. I'm sure you've noticed before if you eat a lot of processed or sugar-rich food, this can influence your energy levels later in the day.

To help us think about how nutrition affects performance, I want to make some distinctions that might be useful. This way you can understand better how what you eat will impact what you can do. You can think of there being three layers to performance:

1. At the most fundamental level, what you eat will affect your **baseline health** and can change your ability to do anything over the course of a long period of time. Diet has been linked to chronic diseases like diabetes, cardiovascular disease, hypertension, stroke and cancer. As we'll see in the next chapter, a plant-based diet is a great start in preventing these conditions.

2. If you're not in a state of ill health, your ability to perform will be dictated largely by your **physical fitness**. This is defined by what you do with your body on a regular basis – how you train it, or don't, the levels of stress in your life, the quality of your sleep and, of course, what you put into it in terms of nutrition. All these factors are interdependent, but at the center is nutrition. It will determine how well you can train, and this will have a knock-on effect to sleep and stress.

3. The third layer is really an extension of the last. If you're not in a state of ill health, and you not only have a reasonable level of physical fitness, but you are also expecting your body to be able to do something more, you can think of this as a kind of **peak performance**. For instance, it could be that you want to run a

marathon, or that you're looking to put on extra lean muscle. It could be that you're an athlete, specializing in a particular sport that needs a specialized kind of training. It could be that you want to optimize your health on all fronts. This is often what I try to work towards with my clients – it gives you a clear route of how to get the most out of life. And this will all need a personalized approach to nutrition.

The information contained within this book will cover how nutrition directly affects all these different areas of performance. Right now, we're going to look at the components of physical fitness.

FITNESS

Physical fitness is multidimensional. It is also relative to the individual: fitness metrics in a 70-year-old looks very different from a 20-year-old. There are clear components that you can work on to improve your fitness at any age, and they all require specific training.

Cardiorespiratory fitness: the ability of your heart and lungs to provide enough oxygen and nutrients to the muscles that need it, when they need it, and to remove carbon dioxide and the other waste products of metabolism. This is what most people think of as fitness: how quickly you run out of gas when going at full tilt. One way of quantifying it is to measure your VO2 max – the maximum amount of oxygen your body can use during exercise.

Muscular strength and endurance: Muscular strength is the ability to exert force against resistance, while muscular endurance is the ability of the muscle or muscle group to exert force repeatedly. Muscular strength isn't solely correlated to the crosssectional size of the muscle. In other words, just because you're bigger doesn't necessarily mean you'll be stronger, although it'd be the obvious bet. Strength is also a function of the nervous system – getting more of the muscle fibers to contract in a coordinated way.

Body composition and flexibility: There are certain activities, like yoga, gymnastics, or dance that require a base level of flexibility to be able to perform them at all. In general, range of movement will define how well any kind of movement can be performed. Think about a golf swing or reaching down to tie your shoelaces. Body composition refers to the varying percentages of muscle, bone, and fat in your body. Two different people can be of a similar height and weight but have very different body compositions.

Balance, agility, and coordination: All three components to physical fitness define your ability to play a sport or execute any kind of movement, whether complex or not, from high level acrobatics and ball-based sports to playing catch or catching something that you've knocked off a table.

Reaction time and power: These are both improvable variables in your physical makeup. Power is usually defined as the ability to use strength at speed, while reaction time is how quickly you respond to a stimulus in the first place.

Recovery: Some sporting activities depend on the ability to recover from recurrent minor injuries – think about the minor (and sometimes not so minor) traumas that you repeatedly receive when you play a contact sport. Operating at a very high level requires a high intensity of training, and this requires the body to recover quickly enough to continue the training within a structured program.

WHERE DOES FOOD COME IN?

You can immediately see that almost everything that constitutes your physical fitness is directly affected by your diet. In order to improve your cardiorespiratory fitness, you need to make sure that you are not eating foods which are damaging to your cardio-vascular system. Then you need to make sure that your body is sufficiently fueled to be able to train this kind of fitness. Muscular strength and endurance will similarly require the right kind of nutrition at the right time to ensure you can train in the right way, and the right kind of food to aid recovery and growth. Body composition, more than anything, is most obviously affected by what you eat. Even aspects which seem unrelated to nutrition like flexibility or balance and coordination, or even power, are all modulated by the nervous system, and we shall see in Chapter 10 that your nervous system is inextricably linked to your digestive system, through the gut-brain axis.

Of course, training will play the deciding role in final outcomes, but I'm breaking down this list to try and emphasize that everything you do is founded on what you eat. Proper nutri-tion forms the basis for your ability to successfully perform all physical activities. It plays a major role in the following aspects:

Muscle maintenance: The muscles are the most significant component of the human body, and they need sufficient nutrition to function well. About 70% of the body is taken up by muscles (more if you're muscly, less if you're less). Muscles are multi-functional. Attached to the bones, they allow both voluntary and involuntary movement in the body. They help regulate body temperature through shivering or sweating when necessary. Furthermore, they assist in the circulation of blood by helping to expand and constrict blood vessels.

To increase muscle mass, you need to be in a caloric surplus, which means that you need to take in more calories than your body uses daily. Additionally, you must consume enough protein in your diet. Protein is the building block for muscles and without it, the body will not be able to properly build and repair muscles after exercise. This becomes particularly important as you age as wear and tear takes its toll. There are abundant amounts of protein available from plant-based sources, but depending on your performance goals, protein can be a complicated subject that we'll look at more closely in Chapter 6.

Bone health: Bones are a type of connective tissue and provide weight and structure to the body. Nutritional deficiencies can weaken bones and lead to skeletal disorders, including a weakened bone structure, a higher risk of fracture, and the development of osteoporosis.[2] To maintain strong, healthy bones, it is important to make sure that you are getting enough calcium and vitamin D in your diet (see Chapter 8). In addition to this, you should ensure that your daily caloric intake is sufficient for maintaining your weight as well as providing support for muscle growth and repair. One of the best ways to keep your bones strong is to keep your whole body strong. This is also particularly important as you age.

Immune function: A diet that lacks essential nutrients will lead to a weakened immune system, which makes it harder for our bodies to fight off infections and illnesses. One of the most important things that you can do for your immunity is to eat well. There are many different ways in which diet affects immunity, but there are some key nutrients that are especially important to ensure it functions at its best.

Vitamin A, found in leafy green vegetables, helps to maintain healthy mucous membranes throughout the body. These membranes line the intestines and lungs, and they also protect against toxins entering the bloodstream via food particles or air pollutants.[3]

Vitamin C, found in citrus fruits, helps to maintain healthy blood cells that fight infection. In fact, a whole range of micronutrients are needed to keep the immune system running properly: vitamins D, E,

B6, and B12, folate, iron, zinc, copper, selenium, and magnesium. Plants contain these in large quantities, and the lists of foods which support your immune system are always topped by plants, like citrus fruits, red peppers, garlic and ginger.

Brain function: The brain requires a large amount of energy for it to work properly. It is the organ with the highest demand for blood in the body. It weighs only 3 pounds (about 1.36 kg) but uses 20% of the oxygen and nutrients carried in the blood. Fueling the brain with proper nutrition will help maintain its optimal performance. It may also benefit from certain foods. For example, omega-3 fatty acids are important for its development and functioning, ensuring normal cognitive development in both children and adults. The right balance of omega-3 fatty acids is also important for preventing neurological disorders like Alzheimer's disease[4] and alleviating ADHD,[5] as well as potentially treating some kinds of depression (more of this in Chapter 8).[6]

Mental and emotional health: Our moods are regulated by two crucial hormones, serotonin and dopamine. Serotonin is made from the essential amino acid tryptophan while dopamine is made from tyrosine, a non-essential amino acid. Studies also show that eating a balanced diet (avoiding processed foods and getting a good quantity of micro-nutrients, in particular magnesium, folic acid and B vitamins) can reduce the risk for depression and anxiety.[7] Specifically, when the body is deficient in these nutrients, it won't be able to produce the right amounts of these hormones which may lead to mood swings and less stable emotional health.[8]

WHAT DO YOU WANT TO DO?

This is the big question to ask yourself in terms of nutrition. *What do you want your diet to support?* If you have specific goals, this can be incredibly motivating to make sure that your diet is as effective as possible in ensuring your success. This will really give you incentive to plan and eat well. Even if your aim is just to stay physically fit, you can see that there are many different dimensions to this endeavor, from cardiorespiratory fitness to reaction time. It provides a great framework for you to plan your training, which needs to be underpinned by a strong nutrition plan. Food will always be fundamental to it all, providing a foundation you can build on. And that's the bottom line, the foundation of health, and that's going to be the subject of the next chapter.

CHAPTER 3

THE POWER OF PLANTS

Nothing will benefit human health and increase the chances for survival of life on Earth as much as the evolution to a vegetarian diet.

Albert Einstein

There's a classic and dismissive saying in the realm of scientific research that "the plural of anecdote isn't data." In other words, when you hear a good story about the effects of something – for instance, the benefits of going plant-based – even when you hear the same kind of story from a whole load of other people, it doesn't count as good scientific evidence. How the stories are collected, who is chosen to tell them, why they've decided to tell them, and all sorts of other factors are involved in making the stories useful as data.

Obtaining good scientific evidence is a rigorous process, and it is especially complicated when it comes to nutrition. Part of the challenge is that it is difficult to set up and conduct big epidemiological studies, which involve large populations and are carried out over many years, often over decades. These are studies which aim to track the prevalence of diseases and health conditions in big groups of people. They can be subject to problems with confounding or self-reporting biases. A self-reporting bias is exactly that – usually people will be biased when reporting about themselves. You can think of confounding as the mixing of effects. For instance, when you can't tell whether someone has good health outcomes because they haven't been eating animal products, or because they are not doing any number of other unhealthy things. When something is considered "healthy," like eating a plant-based diet, the likelihood is that those who follow that healthy diet are also doing other healthy things too, like getting enough exercise and not smoking.

It's much easier to test a drug. You can put it into a randomized double-blind placebo-controlled trial (RCT) and have a much tighter idea of the effects it is having. The problem is that drugs are often not tested against lifestyle interventions. The placebo control will be a sugar pill, rather than a change in diet, and the pharmaceutical industry is much more interested in getting people to buy drugs to control blood pressure or blood sugar rather than have them change the way they eat in the first place.

Of course, there are some RCTs conducted in the field of nutrition – specifically when it comes to testing the components of food and the effects of individual nutrients. Although research generally always has mixed results, there is a growing body of evidence that suggests that switching to a plant-based diet can have a profound effect on some serious health outcomes.

PLANT-BASED DIETS AND CHRONIC DISEASES

This is the big one. The incredible potential impact that plant-based diets might have on chronic disease is often the reason people turn to them to improve their health. Research shows a wide range of benefits that provide protection against diabetes, cardiovascular disease, and cancer; however, researchers do not yet know what exactly causes these benefits. When someone switches to a plant-based diet, there are effectively two different things happening simultaneously. They are reducing the amount of meat, dairy and seafood that they eat, whilst increasing the quantity of fruit and vegetables. It's likely that positive health outcomes are the result of both these actions.

One possible and popular route of explanation is the effect that plant-based diets have on inflammation. Inflammation is a critically important response in the human body when it's faced with injury or infection. However, when it becomes systemic chronic inflammation, it can become the main contributor to the development of these chronic diseases.[1] In very simple terms, plants are rich in phytonutrients and antioxidants, chemicals that help to counter the harmful effects of inflammation, whilst meat tends to be pro-inflammatory.

A large review of research on plant-based diets determined that vegetarian diets are inversely associated with the risk of developing diabetes, and that there is a positive association between eating meat and developing diabetes.[2] Many studies highlight the detrimental effects of eating meat. Its consumption - in particular red meat, processed meat and meat cooked at a high temperature – has been associated with certain kinds of cancer, mainly ones that affect the digestive system, but also prostate cancer as well. This has led the World Health Organization to label processed meat as a Group 1 carcinogen. Bacon-lovers of the world have been up in arms ever since the declaration.

The risk factors for these chronic diseases are often interlinked, so improving one thing can have a positive knock-on effect. For instance, a plant-based diet has been shown to improve blood sugar control[3] and aid in weight loss efforts,[4] which can help to reduce the risk of both diabetes and cardiovascular disease.[5] In an RCT, published in the journal Nutrition and Diabetes, overweight individuals who followed a vegan diet for 16 weeks experienced significant reductions in body weight and insulin resistance compared to the control diet.[6]

PLANT-BASED DIETS AND MORTALITY

What about mortality, the ultimate bottom line? Some research has shown that plant-based eaters actually live longer than people who consume animal products.

A large study that surveyed over 70,000 people determined that vegetarians had a 12% lower risk of mortality than non-vegetarians.[7] Additionally, another study of over 48,000 people found that vegetarians had a 13% lower risk of death from heart disease when compared to meat eaters.[8] Notably though, those who ate fish (but no meat) also had a similar 13% lower risk of death from heart disease. In fact, there are many studies that link a plant-based diet with lower incidence of mortality from cardiovascular disease, and some from all-cause mortality. One from 2016 estimated that replacing just 3% of protein intake from red meat and eggs with plant protein would significantly reduce all-cause mortality.[9]

However, it is worth noting that although some studies show a decrease in death from heart disease on a plant-based diet, the same studies show an increase in the risk of stroke on a plant-based diet when compared to one that includes meat.

So, the evidence is mixed. And it is also prudent to keep in mind that eating plant-based alone doesn't automatically make you live longer. Other factors in your life also play an integral role such as genetics, exercise, adequate sleep, managing stress and avoiding environmental toxins, to name just a few.

PLANT-BASED DIETS AND INFLAMMATORY AND AUTOIMMUNE DISEASES

An autoimmune disease is characterized by the immune system mistakenly attacking the body instead of an invading pathogen. An increasing amount of evidence indicates that many autoimmune diseases can be positively impacted by following a plant-based diet. When individuals refrain from eating meat and dairy products, they have reported a significant reduction - or even a complete reversal - of the symptoms associated with autoimmune disorders.

Depending on which system of the body is under attack and how severe the disorder is, there are around 80 different types of autoimmune disorders. For unknown reasons, women, especially during their childbearing years, are more susceptible to autoimmune conditions than men. Some speculate that sex hormones may contribute to the condition. Generally, autoimmune disorders are incurable, but their symptoms are manageable. The effect of a plant-based diet on autoimmune conditions could be down to the removal of some of the trigger foods, like meat, diary, and eggs, or it could be because of what the plants themselves contain. As we've discussed, foods like olive oil, nuts, and seeds, contain anti-inflammatory compounds.

Rheumatoid arthritis, a condition that affects approximately 1% of the world's population, has shown the most promising research. Studies have shown that removing animal products from the diet reduces rheumatoid arthritis symptoms[10] - that meant a decrease in swollen joints during the time that a vegan diet was followed. There is less research on other autoimmune diseases. For instance, there are many anecdotal examples of people reversing their symptoms of lupus with a plant-based diet (Brooke Goldner, a celebrity doctor and author of Goodbye Autoimmune Disease and Goodbye Lupus is the most notable), but few studies are yet to back up the reports.

PLANT-BASED DIETS AND ATHLETIC PERFORMANCE

Although there is plenty of evidence to suggest that vegetarian or vegan diets protect against chronic diseases such as heart disease, diabetes, and cancer, evidence of the relationship between plant-based diets and performance in exercise capacities among athletes is still pretty limited. More research is needed on this subject. This does not mean that a vegan diet isn't beneficial for athletes, it's just that the evidence-based links are yet to be made.

The following are some potential benefits that may be experienced by athletes consuming a plant-based diet:

Enhanced glucose storage: For aerobic exercise, carbohydrates are the main fuel source. However, many athletes do not consume enough carbohydrates to sustain their active lifestyles. Glucose is stored in the body as glycogen. The body uses glycogen stores from the liver or muscles to produce energy during exercise and they will become depleted if there is not enough carbohydrate intake. One study found that only 46% of endurance athletes consumed enough carbohydrates to train for 1-3 hours per day.[11] As an athlete consuming a plant-based diet, you will likely have higher glycogen stores because legumes, whole grains, and root vegetables are abundant in complex carbohydrates, and will make up the main source of calories in your diet.

Enhanced blood circulation: All athletes' performance is hugely influenced by the circulation of blood, as it transports nutrients, oxygen, and waste gases produced by metabolism to and from the muscles. In this way, arterial health can affect our body's ability to perform these functions, and reduced blood flow will severely negatively affect athletic performance. Plant-based diets reduce blood viscosity, improve the flexibility of the arteries and the functioning of the artery walls which results overall in a better blood flow and oxygenation of all the tissues in the body.[12] Nitrates in the diet may increase blood flow and improve exercise performance and recovery. Nitrates help the body in dilating the arteries and maintaining smooth blood flow. Some foods that contain nitrates, which may benefit the health of your arteries, include beetroot, citrus fruits, watermelon, and green leafy vegetables.[13]

Lower oxidative stress: Free radicals are produced when muscles are put under stress during exercise, in particular when the exercise is exhaustive. Oxidative stress and muscle damage occurs when a body's ability to neutralize free radicals with antioxidants is exceeded by the rate it produces them. A high level of oxidative stress may damage cells (this is one theory of how aging affects the body), increase blood lipid levels, and reduce muscle strength and performance. Research indicates that those who follow a plant-based diet have higher antioxidant activity than people who eat meat because of their high consumption of antioxidants and other phytonutrients which are present in plants, but not in animal products.[14] For instance, vitamin C, which is found abundantly in plants works as an antioxidant in the body.

Decreased inflammation: As we discussed earlier in the chapter, inflammation is known to be associated with chronic diseases, and as well as diet, exercise can help reduce chronic inflammation.[15] However, exercise can also cause short-term inflammation as well. Muscle soreness, slow or impaired recovery post-workout and performance loss are common symptoms. These short-term inflammations cannot be completely prevented, but they should be treated as soon as possible by providing the body with the right nutrients. Anti-inflammatory properties are associated with healthy fats, such as monounsaturated fatty acids and omega-3 fatty acids, which can be found in plants. A meta-analysis of multiple studies determined that over a two-year period, adherence to plant-based diets reduced inflammation.[16]

Recovery: Plant-based diets are not only beneficial for athletes during training and competition, but they can also be helpful for recovery. After a strenuous workout, your body needs time to repair and rebuild damaged muscles. If you don't eat enough nutritious food, you won't recover as quickly from your workouts and may even start to experience negative side effects such as fatigue, illness, and injury. Consuming plenty of protein—which can be found abundantly in a well-planned plant-based diet—will help with this process. Research suggests that plant-based eating can improve endurance athlete's recovery time.[12]

Anecdotally, improved recovery is a big reason why many athletes switch to a vegan or more plant-based diet. Many of my clients often comment on how they feel less of the negative effects of post-workout recovery, like reduced energy levels or muscle soreness, once they've made the change to a plant-based diet.

WHAT'S THE BEST DIET FOR HUMAN HEALTH?

As we discovered in Chapter 1, calling a diet "plant-based" doesn't tell you much more about it than there is a focus on eating plants rather than animal products. Even calling a diet vegan, doesn't tell you exactly what it contains. Two vegan diets can look very different in terms of macronutrient balance and where the calories are coming from, yet still be labelled vegan. As I've said before and I'm always keen to remind my clients, calling yourself vegan doesn't immediately make your diet healthy: you could be getting all your calories from soda, fries and fake meat burgers.

This is where the whole food plant-based (WFPB) diet comes in. It's a dietary pattern that leverages all the advantages of not eating meat, eating more vegetables, and removing processed foods from the diet. People who follow it are often evangelical in praising its benefits. And it's no wonder! The potential benefits are prodigious – increased heart health, reduced cancer risk, slowed cognitive decline, and the prevention of diabetes. In fact, the voices that promote the WFPB diet can be so loud, and our desire to have an unequivocal answer can be so strong, that it might make you feel that it is categorically the best diet for human health.

I definitely don't follow a WFPB diet all the time – I sometimes eat processed foods – but I have on occasion. Anecdotally, I can say that the times that I have been stricter with only eating whole foods, I've felt the physical benefits. I've felt amazing! When everything's on point you feel that you can take on the world. Sometimes I wonder whether the feeling of increased energy and vitality is down to the placebo effect. When eating a WFPB diet, my diet hasn't changed considerably (I still eat exclusively plant-based) but maybe knowing that I'm being extra careful with avoiding added sugars and refined oils, doing all my meal prep, and being on top of my nutrition gives me an extra mental boost. Either way I'll take it!

However, at the moment, there is no research that focuses exclusively on the WFPB diet. The benefits it might give are inferred from research on cutting out animal products and processed foods. And although it might be a diet that has a substantial number of life-changing benefits when looking at statistical averages in large populations, it does not mean that it is necessarily the best diet for you. Or more precisely, everything that falls under the umbrella of a WFPB diet might not be the best food for you, and some of the things that don't (for instance some animal products) might actually be highly beneficial for your own personal health.

In other words, there's no simple answer to the question: "What's the best diet for human health?"

The only reasonable answer is: *it depends.*

Eran Segal, a computational biologist, took a novel approach to better understand the question. He measured "meal glucose response" – the changes in blood sugar levels after eating a meal – in 1,000 people for an entire week, measuring blood glucose levels after every meal. He also tracked exactly what they ate, so that he could connect the measurements to foods. Meal glucose response is an interesting metric to look at, because it has been associated with obesity, diabetes and cardiovascular disease, and higher levels of glucose in the blood after meals is correlated to higher levels of mortality.

What he discovered were trends that you might expect – for instance that eating carbohydrates spiked blood glucose levels. However, what he also found was that these trends weren't universal, that individuals responded very differently to eating the same foods. For instance, some people had spikes in blood glucose after eating ice cream and did not have the same response after eating rice, but for others it was the reverse – blood sugar was spiked by rice, but not by ice cream. In fact, in his data set, the proportion of people in the latter group was higher – rice had a worse effect on blood sugar than ice cream for more people. Probably not the result you were expecting![17]

Ultimately individual responses to diet are exactly that – individual. So, it's impossible to settle on a "best" diet for human health, even if the WFPB diet seems like a very good candidate. You have to make it the best diet for you, which means further selection within the foods available from the diet you choose. In other words, if you want to go plant-based, make sure that the foods you're eating from the plant-based diet are optimal for you.

Meal glucose response is only one dimension of health. There are many other important ones, like blood pressure, cholesterol levels and arterial function. It definitely informs on a very important part of long-term health which has a profound impact on performance, and it is a very responsive variable to measure. If you are interested in what particular foods spike your blood glucose more than others, you can now buy affordable home testing kits which make it easier to monitor – you'll probably be surprised by which foods affect you most.

I really believe that there is a tremendous benefit to feeling that you are doing the best you can. You can look at your diet as a process that can be systematically optimized. Start with a practical framework – the WFPB diet for instance – and work from there. Don't get stuck on a principle – get involved with what actually works for your body. This is the long-term approach but helps ensure that you'll be around for the long term.

CHAPTER 4

TRAILBLAZERS & GAME CHANGERS

I've found that a person does not need protein from meat to be a successful athlete. In fact, my best year of track competition was the first year I ate a vegan diet.

Carl Lewis

The legendary track and field athlete Carl Lewis turned to a plant-based diet fairly late in his career. He decided that in order to stay in the game, he had to change the way he ate. He has won nine Olympic gold medals and ten world championships during his distinguished track and field career, making him one of the top athletes of the last century. When he set the world record for the 100-meter dash, he did it when he was 30 years old having just switched to a plant-based diet. And this was back in the 1990s when veganism was far from mainstream.

It's old news now that the diet of Roman gladiators, whose lives depended on their athletic performance, was predominantly plant-based. It's also not entirely accurate. They did eat a lot of plants, and so much barley that they gained the nickname hordearii ("barley-eaters"), but analysis of their bones reveals they also ate some meat and fish. In the past, they have been used as the poster boys for a plant-based diet, a way to convince the men who believe that masculinity is only associated with eating red meat that eating plants doesn't make you any less of a man.

Famous athletes and sports personalities changing to a plant-based or vegan diet always make the headlines, and that's only partly because of our culture's fascination with the private life of celebrities (for instance, Wikipedia has its own page, "List of vegans" which is just a list of celebrities who are vegan). It's also because at this point in the 21st century, it's still challenging convention. For so long animal products have been at the center of human nutrition. It's amazing to see that the peak of human endeavor can be achieved without relying on the life of another species. It's clear that meat does not give you a competitive advantage.

IT DOESN'T MATTER WHAT YOU DO

It doesn't matter what domain you're expert in, every sport has professional vegan players, from soccer and American football players to strongmen, tennis players, snowboarders and cyclists. Today, there are so many successful athletes who follow a plant-based diet and they do it for all of the reasons we covered in the last chapter: improved health, reduced inflammation, and faster recovery time.

Some high-profile examples include:

Lewis Hamilton went plant-based in 2018 to improve his energy levels and as he became more conscious of the environmental impact of eating animal products. Hamilton says he feels more focused now that he's on the diet, sleeps better, and recovers quicker. The only regret he has is not having started eating plant-based sooner.

Tia Blanco is a professional surfer, one of the best on the planet, world champion in 2015 and 2016. Blanco attributes her decision to go vegan to her love of and appreciation of the environment. Her evident level of fitness and accomplishments in such a challenging sport makes it difficult to claim that she hasn't benefited from a plant-based diet.

Scott Jurek, an award-winning and record-breaking athlete from Duluth, Minnesota, has competed in Ultramarathons on a plant-based diet since 1999. He is one of the world's best ultramarathoners and holds the record for the longest distance run in 24 hours (165.7 miles). He explains his transition into veganism in his autobiography, Eat & Run, that the plant-based diet has been an important part of his journey.

Novak Djokovic hasn't eaten meat for many years. In 2010, he became vegetarian and the turnaround in his dietary choices began when his nutritionist discovered he had a gluten sensitivity and recommended eliminating gluten and dairy. In the following years, he eliminated all animal products from his diet and attributes his impressive performance and recovery to eating plant based. Since 2011, his career has risen to new heights and today he is regarded as one of the greatest tennis players of all time.

The list could go on and on, and it's only increasing as more world-class athletes join the ranks of plant-based eaters. At the moment, they are trailblazers, but hopefully it will just become the norm and it'll no longer make the news that celebrated athletes are vegan.

Also, given time, we might get a better understanding of how eating a plant-based diet effects the entire life span of a world-class athlete. So far, the examples we've given have been of those who've become vegan in adulthood.

PLANT-BASED EATING FOR CHILDREN: SHOULD YOU START THEM YOUNG?

When you see someone like Patrik Baboumian carrying a yoke round his shoulders with 4 people balanced on it, your first thought is – he's incredibly strong. And you'd be right, he's a strongman and former body builder. And, unusually, he's also a vegan. Your next thought might then be, "When did he go vegan?"

Baboumian hasn't been vegan his whole life, but went vegetarian when he was almost 30, and vegan a few years after. He certainly shows that it's possible to be vegan and to be incredibly strong. He also raises the interesting question of whether it's possible to grow up as a vegan and to achieve a similar level of performance. What if you ate a vegan diet from day one?

From my personal experience, most of the "gainz" that I made, my biggest relative increases in size and mass, were when I was on a diet that included a large amount of animal protein. That was from when I was first born, until late adolescence. In particular, I feel I laid the foundation for the body I have now when I was a teenager. At the time I ate the usual amount of hamburgers and milkshakes that American teenagers ate in the 1980s. It's impossible to know what I'd be like if I'd been vegan from day one, just like it's impossible to know whether the athletes who are now plant-based would be capable of the same kind of performance if they had grown up eating a plant-based diet. It's an important question to consider because more and more vegan parents are bringing up their children on a purely plant-based diet. Would

Djokovic have won 17 grand slams if he'd learnt to play tennis while only eating plants?

Purely from the perspective of overall health, a plant-based diet from a young age appears to confer notable benefits. Research suggests that eating plant-based diets early on can prevent heart disease later in life since plaque buildup in the arteries starts in childhood.[1] There may also be some association between dairy consumption during childhood and the risk of prostate cancer as an adult.[2] Moreover, children who consume a plant-based diet are likely to have a lower incidence of obesity and are less likely to be overweight.[3]

Despite the fact that plant-based diets have been proven to be safe and healthy, a lot of critics maintain that children shouldn't be excluded from eating animal products altogether, due to the nutrients that might be missing from the diet (as we shall cover in Chapter 8). Critical periods of development need optimal nutrition.

However, there is research which supports plant-based diets from a macronutrient point of view. A 2019 study conducted in Germany compared energy intake and macronutrient intake among children from ages 1 to 3 who followed a vegan, vegetarian, or omnivorous diet. According to the researchers, an omnivorous diet tends to be higher in protein and sugar, while a vegan diet tends to be higher in carbohydrates and fiber, although both diets had above the recommended levels of protein. Their study found that plant-based diets can support normal growth patterns while meeting the nutritional needs of children.[4]

Although this is a great study suggesting some interesting outcomes, especially because it covers such a young age group, there are a couple of things to bear in mind. Firstly, it was quite small, with only 127 vegan children. It was also a cross-sectional study, which means it was an observational study that takes a cross section through a population at a particular moment in time, relying on data that might be provided by the participants and therefore suffer from reporting errors or recall bias. Secondly, a slightly larger number of the children in the vegan group suffered from stunted growth compared to the omnivorous group which the researchers determined was down to getting insufficient calories. This is an issue we will discuss in the next chapter – making sure that your energy input is adequate for the output you're expecting – and can be more of a problem on a vegan diet because plants are often less energy dense, but more filling than animal products.

REPORTING NUTRITION CLAIMS: A PROBLEM OF BIAS

As with any diet, there are always going to be people who swear by its benefits and those who are skeptical of its claims. This is especially true when it comes to diets that challenge the status quo, like plant-based ones.

One group that vocally opposes the vegan diet is the proponents of what are often termed "ancestral" diets. This can include paleo, or Primal, or similar variations, where eating locally sourced unprocessed whole foods in a pattern similar to how ancestral humans might have eaten is emphasized. I say "might" because the paleo diet bears no real resemblance to how paleolithic humans would have eaten. Organic meat and forageable food (like berries and leafy greens) rather than the products of modern agriculture (like grains) are at the forefront. The argument goes that because humans have always been omnivorous, it will be impossible to achieve peak performance unless following the dietary pattern that has been established by countless generations of human evolution.

It's very easy to find good research that backs up parts of this argument, just like I have found good research to back up the proposal that following a plant-based diet will lead to positive health outcomes that won't be experienced when eating animal products. You can always find research or use statistics to substantiate a claim, and you can usually always find problems with the research that an opposing opinion uses to make their own arguments. This isn't to say that you can't believe anything you read, but that you should be aware of the bias that a claim comes with and understand that it will affect the message that it is endorsing.

It's certainly true of claims for the benefits of ancestral diets – they tend to play down parts of the research that are negative towards dietary saturated fats and cholesterol. But it's also true of claims for the benefits of vegan diets as well.

For example, *The Game Changers* is a documentary from 2018 that extols the benefits of plant-based eating for athletes. The film follows a number of athletes who have made the switch to a plant-based diet and showcases their success in various sports.

On one level it was a great film because it brought a positive message about plant-based eating to the mainstream and encouraged people to believe in their capabilities, regardless of the diet they're eating. However, from early on, you can clearly see that the film is only telling one side of the story and has a noticeably clear research bias. It uses weak or unscientific studies and completely ignores the research that suggests some forms of animal products might provide some health benefits to some people, whilst making claims that can't really be substantiated – like that a plant-based diet will definitely result in superior athletic performance to one that contains meat.

Because the film came across so clearly as a kind of vegan propaganda, and because of the potential connections between some of the people involved in the film and the plant-based food industry, there was an enormous backlash on the internet, with multiple articles and videos debunking the pro-vegan claims made in the film. Ultimately this type of thing can end up damaging the message that veganism is trying to spread, the kind of message I hope this book will proliferate.

I wanted to include a chapter that mentioned athletes who are currently performing at world-class levels on a vegan diet, not as proof that a vegan diet will make you athletically superior, but as motivation and inspiration. Ultimately, I want to present an unbiased view of a plant-based diet, so that you can make the best choices for your personal needs. I hope you will understand that your personal needs are tied to the needs of the planet and all the beings that inhabit it. And I want you to understand the challenges you will face, just as much as the benefits you can receive.

Nutrition takes work, first in understanding what you need, and then in implementing it. The second part is up to you, but I hope I can help with the first part. In the next few chapters, we will do exactly that – look in depth at plant-based nutrition. This will provide you with the blueprint for working out what you need.

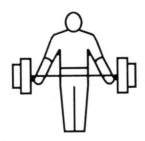

CHAPTER 5

FOOD IS FUEL

Food is fuel and it keeps us going just like a car needs petrol. When you're running a car it's important to think about what fuel you're putting in because if you put in the rough stuff, what's going to happen? The car's going to slow down and perform badly because you've neglected it.

William Katt

For some people, food is just that: fuel. A means of providing your body with the nutrients and energy it needs to keep your heart pumping, your brain alert, and your muscles firing. For others, it is a way of connecting with other people, a way of expressing themselves creatively and identifying with their culture. It can be all these things if you want it to! By all means do your weekly food prep, plan your pre- and post-workout meals, count your macros and fuel your body sufficiently, but don't lose sight of how important food is as part of the human social experience.

The cliché that "food is fuel" is actually only true to a certain extent. The macronutrients in food provide calories, which the body uses for energy. As we discussed in Chapter 1, food also contains important micronutrients and phytochemicals which are vital for supporting the health of your body, but don't supply any energy in themselves. This is one of the big benefits of eating plants: fruit and vegetables contain these in abundance. Food fulfills a complex role, delivering messages to all different parts of your body, influencing levels of hormones and neurotransmitters, all of which have an impact on how your body can perform. A piece of food goes through a complex journey as it goes in one end and out the other!

In this chapter we're going to look at how food provides energy for your body, concentrating in particular on carbohydrates, one of the biggest sources of energy in a plant-based diet.

HOW MUCH ENERGY DO YOU NEED IN A DAY?

Energy requirements vary dramatically for different people. Depending on what you're doing in the day, you're going to need more or less fuel to keep yourself going. If you spend all day sitting down (highly unrecommend!), then you'll need less input than if you are training hard. This is obvious enough. You need to eat enough calories to fuel whatever you're doing. Data points towards a lower overall energy consumption in vegans as opposed to omnivores.[1]

You burn calories from performing any activity, but you also burn them just by being alive. The number of calories you burn without any activity is called your basal metabolic rate (BMR). It's determined by a variety of factors, including age, height, gender and weight.[2] To calculate your daily calorie needs, you also need to estimate your total daily energy expenditure (TDEE) - a multiplier that takes into account your activity levels.

The original calculations for BMR were done in 1919 by Harris and Benedict and are often called the Harris-Benedict principle. They have since been updated several times, and to calculate your BMR, you can use the following formulas[3]:

▶ **MEN**: BMR = 10 x weight (kg) + 6.25 x height (cm) – 5 x age (years) + 5

▶ **WOMEN**: BMR = 10 x weight (kg) + 6.25 x height (cm) – 5 x age (years) - 161

For example, I'm a 47-year-old man who is 187cm tall (about 6'1") and at the moment I'm on the light side and weigh 85kg (187 lb).

My BMR is 10 x 85 + 6.25 x 187 - 5 x 47 + 5 = 1,789 kcal

Aisha, my co-author, on the other hand, is 35-year-old woman who is 160cm tall (about 5'3") and weighs 61 kg (134 lb).

She has a BMR of 10 x 61 + 6.25 x 160 – 5 x 35 - 161 = 1,274 kcal

To calculate your TDEE, multiply your BMR by a physical activity level[4]:

- If you are sedentary (little or no exercise): BMR x 1.2
- If you are lightly active (light exercise/sports 1-3 days/week): BMR x 1.375
- If you are moderately active (moderate exercise/sports 3-5 days/week): BMR x 1.55
- If you are very active (heavy exercise/sports 6-7 days a week): BMR x 1.725
- If you are extra active (very heavy exercise/sports and physical job or 2x training): BMR x 1.9
- If you are a professional athlete: BMR x 2.4

For example, I'm extra active – I train by lifting weights every day (apart from my scheduled rest days), and often when I train my clients, I'll run with them, or do something equally active to keep them motivated. My total daily energy expenditure would be:

1,789 x 1.9 = 3,399 kcal

Aisha is a moderately active, she sometimes goes running and practices yoga and HIIT during the week, so her TDEE would be:

1,274 kcal x 1.55 = 1,975 kcal

Calculating your TDEE gives you a rough figure of how many calories you burn in a day. Nowadays it's easier to get much more granular with exactly how many calories you're using because smart watches and other devices can track and log exactly how much energy was expended from activity to activity. If you have the equipment and inclination, it's well worth recording exactly how much energy you use on a day-to-day basis. Unless you're working towards a particular training goal it can get a bit tedious to do it all the time, but if you record a couple of weeks and take an average, it will give you a more accurate idea of your energy expenditure over a week, based on the activities you are regularly doing.

The most notable factor is that BMR changes with age: it goes down. So, as you get older, you'll need to consume fewer calories. One reason this occurs could be to do with changes in body composition. Although BMR is calculated by weight, what is really significant is fat-free mass – it's the muscles which burn the calories. As you get older, fat-free mass tends to go down. You lose muscle and even though your weight might increase, it's usually from increased fat. This also means that if you are carrying a lot of extra body fat, you need to adjust your BMR calculation to take this into account. There are numerous ways to calculate your percentage body fat, and you can always get a personal trainer or healthcare professional to help you if you're not sure how.

CHANGING YOUR BODY COMPOSITION

Many of the people I've worked with throughout my career have wanted to change their body composition in some way. Some, of course, have had very specific training goals in mind related to their particular athletic endeavor, and any changes in muscle mass or body fat percentage has been collateral to that. Many people who work with a trainer either want to bulk up or lose weight. Putting on weight is usually easier – in very simple terms, do heavy resistance training and eat more, especially protein. Losing weight can be more complex.

In order to lose weight, you need to be in a calorie deficit – you need to eat less calories than you are burning. Some research suggests that the method of weight loss (diet or exercise) isn't important, just that your energy requirements are greater than consumption.[5] The best way to do this is through managing your diet in combination with making sure you are physically active throughout the week. However, it is important to note that weight loss is often a little bit more complicated than just calories in vs calories out. There are a number of factors that can affect your ability to lose weight, including hormones, metabolism, and genetics.[6]

UNDERSTANDING WEIGHT LOSS BEYOND 'CALORIES IN VS CALORIES OUT'

The idea that if you wish to lose weight, you must consume fewer calories than you expend is easy to understand. The extra calories which you eat are stored for future use once your body's energy needs have been met - some as glycogen in muscles and the liver and most as fat in the body. It seems like a simple equation. However, while it is true that the "calories in vs. calories out" model can be helpful for weight loss, it does come with certain limitations. As always with nutrition, it's more complex: different foods have different effects on different processes in the body despite having the same calorie content.

For instance, your metabolism is affected differently by the things you eat. Digestion, absorption, or metabolization of some foods requires more effort than others. The thermic effect of food (TEF) is used to quantitate this work.[7] An item of food requires more energy to be metabolized if it has a high TEF. Proteins have the highest TEF, whereas fats have the lowest. In other words, a high-protein diet requires the body to burn more calories than a high-fat diet. The consumption of protein thus improves your metabolism more significantly than the consumption of carbohydrates or fat.

Notably, 'calories in vs calories out' also fails to account for nutrient density, which gives it limited credibility regarding health. As we discussed in Chapter 1, the nutritional content of foods can vary greatly, independent of their calorie content. Remember, nutrient-dense foods contain higher levels of vitamins, minerals, and other constituents per gram. An apple and a chocolate chip cookie may contain the same number of calories, and the apple may even contain more sugar than the cookie in some cases, but everything is delivered in a different format. The apple contains fiber and a much higher level of vitamins, minerals, and healthy plant compounds than the cookie. This will mean that regular consumption of apples will have more positive downstream effects than the eating cookies, which will change the conditions for weight gain or weight loss in the body. A lot of this process is modulated by hormones.

HOW FULL DO YOU FEEL?

The nutrients you consume affect your hunger and fullness levels. If you eat 200 calories of nutrient-dense beans, you'll feel much less hungry than if you eat 200 calories of energy-dense chocolate. Foods high in protein and fiber are more filling than those containing relatively small amounts of them.[8] This has a knock-on effect. Because the chocolate is not high in fiber or protein and you don't feel full, you are more likely to overeat later in the day, which increases the odds that you will eat more calories than you need.

Feelings of fullness are affected by what you eat, but feelings of hunger are regulated by hormones. For instance, leptin is a hormone that regulates both appetite and metabolism – sometimes it's called the satiety hormone. If you spend a long time in a calorie deficit, levels of leptin will drop. Your body is responding to the decrease in energy input as a kind of survival mechanism and as a result you will feel hungrier and more tired. Your body is trying to conserve energy and push you into finding more to eat.

In a different pathway, consuming foods high in fructose rather than glucose increases levels of the hunger hormone ghrelin whilst also lowering levels of leptin. It does not activate the same part of the brain that is responsible for regulating fullness as glucose, so when you eat fructose, you won't feel as full especially when the food doesn't contain fiber or protein.[9]

It is well worth remembering that the more processed foods you consume, the harder it is for your hormones to maintain an energy balance, especially when you are deprived of satiating nutrients like protein and fiber. At the end of Chapter 3, we looked at meal glucose response and how it was different for different foods for different people, and this is well worth remembering. Your tastes, your habits, your biochemistry, your gut microbiome, everything about you is unique to you. How food affects you and can change your body composition will also be unique to you.

THE MYTH OF THE 3,500-CALORIE DEFICIT A WEEK

Apart from its fundamental intuitiveness, part of the reason that the idea of 'calories in vs calories out' seems so persuasive as an idea comes down to research that was conducted in the 1950s. Max Wishnofsky determined that losing one pound (0.45kg) of fat per week would require eating approximately 3,500 fewer calories a week.[10] It became a convenient estimate that got absorbed into the advice offered by experts everywhere, from nutritionists to health-focused websites. However, it does not account for the different ways that our bodies process and store calories, how our bodies respond to certain foods, and the overall effects of the endocrine system. A lot of the time, people drastically overestimate their ability to lose weight in a short timeframe.[11]

You could find that in the first week of a diet with 3,500-calorie deficit, you might well lose a pound of fat, but that it doesn't last. As your bodyweight reduces, your muscles actually begin to work more efficiently and use fewer calories than before while performing the same amount of work.[12] Changes in energy expenditure will be further compounded if there is loss of muscle mass along with the loss of fat. This will further the reduction in the calories you burn – BMR will lower too as it is associated with fat-free mass. The scientific term for this is "adaptive thermo-genesis," colloquially known as starvation mode.[13] Overall, it is difficult to lose weight in a linear manner, and it has a tendency to slow down as time goes on when you are on a caloric-deficit diet.[14]

So, if you're trying to lose weight, rather than focusing on a specific number, it is more important to maintain a calorie deficit that is sustainable for you and will help you reach your goals. Also, if you spend a long time in a calorie deficit, it's a good idea to take breaks from it every so often. Try taking one week off for every 6-8 weeks you follow a reduced calorie intake. This can have the effect of resetting hormone levels and help break the monotony of a diet. Taking a long-term approach will be more likely to lead to good results.

WHERE DO THE CALORIES COME FROM?

Every piece of food you eat contains energy, and the exact quantity is determined by the different proportion of macronutrients it contains.

Macronutrients are the major class of nutrients that you probably learnt about in school, and they include proteins, carbohydrates, and fats. The calories they contain are as follows:

- Carbohydrate: 4 calories per gram
- Protein: 4 calories per gram
- Fat: 9 calories per gram

How much you eat of each macronutrient will depend on your performance goals, and the specifics of the diet that you are following. For the general population, the American Academy of Nutrition and Dietetics (AND) recommends that 45-65% of our calories come from carbohydrates, 10-35% from proteins, and 20-35% from fats.[15]

However, it's important to keep in mind that these recommendations are quite broad. They are based on averages and may not be right for everyone. For example, if you are very active, you may need more carbohydrates than the AND recommends. If you are looking to put on lean muscle mass, you might need more protein. Or, if you have a medical condition, you may need to adjust your macronutrient percentages according to your treatment protocol. In that kind of situation, it's important to work with a professional who can help you create a plan that is tailored to your individual needs.

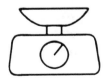

We're going to finish this chapter by concentrating on the primary fuel source for the body:

CARBOHYDRATES

Carbohydrates provide our bodies with fuel for movement and growth. They come in three main types: sugar, starch and fiber. There are many types of sugar including table sugar (sucrose), fruit sugar (fructose) and also the sugar you find in milk (lactose). They are often called simple carbs. Starch is the main form of energy storage in plants, consisting of chains of glucose molecules, often called complex carbs. The form of carbohydrates that is not digestible in the body is known as fiber.

Carbohydrates are produced by plants through the process of photosynthesis, so they are found in the greatest quantities in plants: grains, legumes, fruits, and vegetables. However, these molecules can also be manufactured by animals when they digest their food; this is why carbohydrates can be found to some extent in most of the foods that we eat.

The guidelines recommend that we get about half of our calories from carbohydrates. So, for me that would be about 1,700 kcal. For moderately active Aisha it would be about 988 kcal. That's about 247g of carbohydrates. According to the Institute of Medicine in the US, the recommendation for a completely sedentary adults is only 130g of carbohydrates a day.[16] A single big mac meal contains more carbs than that.

To put that into real food terms, a 2oz (56g) serving of uncooked pasta is about 220 calories. It contains about 42g of carbohydrates, which equates to more than 160 calories. If Aisha ate 6 servings of pasta (and nothing else with it!) she'd have eaten as many carbohydrates as the guidelines recommend for someone her age and size to eat in a day. If she ate 9 bananas, she'd be at her carb limit. That seems like a lot of just pasta or bananas, but remember, everything contains carbs. You're unlikely to eat 9 bananas on their own, but if you're counting your macros to stay with a plan, you've got to pay attention to all the sources.

And carbohydrates are critical for performance. These are their functions in the body[17]:

- A source of energy - the brain, central nervous system, muscles, and red blood cells utilize glucose as their preferred energy source.

- Energy storage - glycogen which is the storage form of glucose is stored in the muscle and liver for use at a later time after a period of fasting.
- Digestion - fiber helps promote regular bowel movements.
- Gives you a feeling of fullness - fiber helps satisfy your hunger after meals and keeps you satisfied for a long time.

In recent years, carbohydrates have come under fire and are often seen as the villain in our attempts to eat a healthy diet, especially if you're trying to manage your weight. There have been countless iterations of low-carb or carb-free diets released onto the market under different brand names. Although, as we shall see below, there are definite concerns over the source of carbohydrates, for most people they remain an essential part of a healthy diet. Unless you're looking into using a different fuel source (see 'The ketogenic diet' in Chapter 7), without sufficient carbohydrates in our diets we would find it hard to get through our workout routines effectively or even perform our daily tasks. Eating them supports key bodily functions such as brain activity, the immune system, and hormone regulation.

If you're an athlete, and you are engaging in high volumes of intense exercise – 8 or more hours a week – you must continually replace the glycogen that your body is using to generate energy in the muscles. The International Society of Sports Nutrition recommends a high daily diet of carbohydrates: 8-12g/kg/day.[18] According to these recommendations, I would need to eat 680-1,020 grams a day, which is way more than the standard 425g a day (at 50% of calorie intake), and definitely more than I currently eat. When I was training for the Ironman, I ate that kind of volume and it meant I spent a large proportion of my day eating!

FUEL SOURCES: THE BODY'S ENERGY SYSTEMS

Resting burns a lot of energy. In fact, between 50-80% of our daily energy is consumed just in the resting state. Eating does too - the very process by which we bring energy into the body, eating, digesting and metabolizing food all burn energy. And when we want to put in the work, we need extra energy, and this is why you need to eat enough carbs to perform well.

To get a good understanding of why carbohydrates are important, we're going to briefly look at the body's energy systems. Bear in mind that this is a broad overview – once you get into the details, the biochemistry gets increasingly complicated.

First, we need to briefly understand the way energy is produced and stored. Muscles use molecules of adenine triphosphate (ATP) to generate contractions, which is why ATP is commonly referred to as the body's energy unit. Active muscles require a constant supply of ATP, and molecules of ATP are also used and replaced every 2 minutes at rest. During intense exercise, this turnover rate can increase by 1,000-fold. In a whole day you go through 50-75kg of ATP, even though there is only 100g of it stored in the body.

ATP is produced through the oxidation of fatty acids from the blood and triglycerides stored in the muscles, and also from blood glucose (there's about 4g of glucose circulating in the bloodstream at any one time) and stores of glycogen in the muscles. Glycogen is also stored in the liver (about 80g), and it's released into the bloodstream at the same rate that the cells take up glucose from the blood. By far the biggest storage of glycogen is in the skeletal muscles (the total weight of glycogen in the body is 600g), and it has the potential to provide the most fuel for the body's energy systems.

In simple terms, there are three energy systems in the body. For a quick burst of energy, the body uses phosphocreatine, a chemical which is stored in the muscles and can quickly replenish the ATP. This energy system is short-lived and can only generate about 10 seconds worth of energy before the fuel is used up. The second system is the glycolytic system, which essentially runs on the breakdown of glucose or glycogen through a series of controlled reactions within the cells. One of the main disadvantages of this system is that it can produce lactic acid, which you feel as a burning sensation in the muscles. Glycolysis doesn't last that long either – only about 2 to 3 minutes.

What is important to note is that the first two systems are anaerobic. That means they can produce energy without oxygen involved in the reactions. The third system is the aerobic one, and in this system all the macronutrients, carbohydrates, fats and even protein can be broken down to produce energy, all using oxygen. If the exercise intensity isn't too high (about 60-80% of VO2 max), this system can last for a long time. It allows the first two systems to get back online, replenishing stores of ATP and phospho-creatine, and clearing the lactic acid. In this third system, carbohydrates are still the most efficient source of fuel, because both protein and fat must go through additional processing before they can be used to produce ATP.

However, one final note that you might find surprising is that carbohydrate is not considered an essential nutrient. These are the nutrients that are needed for the body to function normally that cannot be produced by the body. They consist of 9 amino acids, 2 fatty acids, some vitamins and minerals, but not carbohydrates. All the glucose that your body needs can theoretically be manu-factured by the body.

WHOLE CARBS VS REFINED

Not all carbohydrates are equal. Carbohydrate-containing foods come in many varieties, and their effects on the body vary substantially. The main distinction is between "whole carbs" and "refined carbs."

Whole carbs are those which have undergone minimal processing and still contain the fiber found naturally in the food. Refined carbs have been significantly processed and have lost or changed their natural fiber as well as much of the nutrient content. Think of the difference between brown rice and white rice, or wholegrain bread and white bread. In the refined version of these grains, the bran (the hard outer layer containing fiber, minerals and antioxidants) and the germ (the highly nutrient-rich core of the grain) have been removed, leaving only the endosperm which consists of starchy carbs and protein. All the carbohydrates that food manufacturers add to make foods more palatable are refined carbs – usually simple sugars refined from corn or other plants containing high levels of carbohydrate.

The most basic but best advice for carbohydrate consumption is hopefully something you've heard many times before. Try and get most of your carbohydrate intake from whole carbs: rolled oats, whole grains, barley, legumes, quinoa, beans, and vegetables. Avoid refined carbs where possible: sugary soda, fruit juice, white bread, cakes, pastries, chocolate, and fast food. Here, the simplicity of the whole food diet wins out.

It has been well established that the consumption of refined carbohydrates is linked to several health conditions including obesity and type 2 diabetes.[19] Blood sugar spikes caused by refined carbohydrates can lead to a subsequent crash that triggers hunger and can lead to food cravings.[20] Many essential nutrients are also lacking in refined carbohydrates, which is why they are often labelled "empty" calories. There is also overwhelming evidence that a diet high in added sugar increases the risk of many chronic diseases.[21,22]

Americans tend to eat a lot of added sugar, and most of the rest of the world isn't far behind. To prevent serious health conditions, the US government has recommended that the maximum intake of calories from added sugars should be less than 10% of total calories. However, in my opinion, if you're eating that much added sugar, you're likely to be in line for some sort of health problem down the track. For instance, according to these guidelines, Aisha on her 2,232 calories a day could eat up to 223 calories worth of added sugar, which is the equivalent of 55g or 14 teaspoons of sugar. I could have more than 20 teaspoons – which is a lot! The America Heart Association takes a more conservative approach, limiting energy intakes from added to sugars to just 150 calories for most men (about 9 tsp), and 100 calories for most women (about 6 tsp). If you're under 18, it should be at the low end: not more than 24g (6 tsp) of added sugars per day.

In general, you don't need to worry so much about eating the carbohydrates that come from whole foods. They don't have any added sugars. They are packed with vitamins and other micronutrients, and the fiber they contain means that they do not cause the same blood sugar spikes and dips as refined carbs do. The intake of fiber-rich foods, including vegetables, fruits, legumes,[23] nuts,[24] and whole grains,[25] have been shown in studies to prevent the risk of chronic diseases and improve quality of life.

If we go back to the pasta example above, the 2oz (56g) serving was for pasta made with white flour. An equivalent 2oz serving of whole wheat pasta contains less calories, only 174, and also less carbohydrates – 37g (compared to 42g). The missing weight of carbs is due to an increase in fiber from 2.5g in white pasta to 6g in whole wheat pasta (see below how important fiber is for long-term health). Not only that, but the balance of micronutrients is hugely different. One single serving of whole wheat pasta contains 97% of your recommended daily intake of manganese, an essential mineral important in forming connective tissue and bones, compared with 23% from refined pasta.

HOW QUICK IS THE SUGAR HIT: GLYCEMIC INDEX

As well as classifying carbohydrates by whether they have been refined or not, they can also be categorized by how quickly they raise blood sugar levels. This is their glycemic index (GI). Understanding this will have a big effect on your baseline health if you are trying to manage your blood sugar levels.

Foods are classified as low, medium or high, depending on their score out of 100:

- Low: 55 or less
- Medium: 56–69
- High: 70 or above

Foods that are easy to digest and contain a lot of sugars have a high GI, foods with high protein, fat and fiber content have a low GI. Some foods, like nuts and seeds, have a GI of 0 because what little carbohydrate they consist of is fiber.

It's worth remembering that some foods that have proven health benefits – like whole grains – might have a high GI and you will need to take this into consideration if you're trying to manage blood sugar levels. For instance, white bread has a high GI of 75, which you'd expect, but whole wheat bread isn't much lower, at 74 – also a high GI.

There is a clear positive association between eating foods with a high GI and increasing incidence of type 2 diabetes.[26] However, there is also a time when eating food with a high GI is appropriate. For instance, when you're refueling during heavy training or competition and need to replenish muscle glycogen stores fast.

YOU KNOW IT'S GOOD FOR YOU: FIBER

One major benefit of eating plants is that they contain a lot of fiber, and there is plenty of evidence that eating fiber-rich food will have positive long-term health outcomes. Here's why.

Fiber cannot be completely broken down by the enzymes found in the digestive tract, so it simply passes through it and out of your body without providing you with energy. It can be characterized by how soluble it is, and also by how viscous it is and how easily it ferments. The different types of fiber found in a plant-based diet have different effects on the body – not all fiber acts in the same way.

Fiber, especially the fermentable kind, is an important source of nutrition for many of the organisms in the gut microbiome. A fiber-rich diets can help maintain a diverse microbiome by promoting the growth of these organisms. We'll cover this in more detail in Chapter 10.

Soluble fiber, which is often viscous, absorbs water and slows the movement of food through the digestive system. This delays gastric emptying – food leaving the stomach and entering the small intestine – which increases feelings of fullness and decreases appetite. The result is that fewer calories are consumed, which can result in weight loss (this action is particularly noticeable in overweight populations)[27]. Furthermore, there is both some evidence that eating this kind of fiber can reduce the spikes in blood sugar levels you normally see after eating a meal that is high in carbohydrates, and also that eating it lowers levels of LDL cholesterol in the blood (see Chapter 7 to understand why this is good). The end result is a reduction in the risk for type 2 diabetes and cardiovascular disease. Eating fiber-rich foods also decreases the risk of colon cancer.

Of course, fiber also does exactly what you expect fiber to do: it reduces constipation. Again, the type of fiber makes a difference. Soluble fiber generally increases the bulk of the stool and speeds up its movement through the intestines. Some insoluble fiber will have a similar effect: if it's coarsely ground, it will irritate the large intestine and cause it to secrete water and mucus, which will have the same effect as soluble fiber. If it's finely ground, however, the effect can be the opposite.

An adequate intake has been set by the Institute of Medicine in the US of 38g for an adult male, and 25g for an adult female. If you eat a WFPB diet, you will likely have little problem reaching that target.

CHEAT DAYS

If you're on a strict nutrition plan and you decide on one day of the week not to follow it, it's often referred to as a 'cheat day.' Some trainers swear by them and say that they're the best way for their clients to stick with the diet the rest of the time.

To me, it's a bit like the label "clean eating." It implies a judgement that can often make you feel worse, and although I may occasionally indulge in "cheat days," I never call them that. For a start, I usually try and make sure that I don't eat badly for the whole day – so it's more like a cheat meal! And I don't refer to it as cheating. I call it a celebration. It's a celebration for whatever reason - because it actually is someone's birthday or wedding, or party, or you're celebrating the effort you put in, or the outcomes you've achieved.

Remember, the 'food is fuel' metaphor only gets you so far. The body isn't really like a car: the fuel you put affects all sorts of processes, not just how far it can run. That means food affects every aspect of health, including mental health. Having a healthy mental attitude to food is really important. It's not just energy, it's the very material that you're made of. In the next chapter, we're going to look at protein, the material that constructs so much of what your body consists of.

CHAPTER 6

PROTEIN: WHEN ENOUGH IS ENOUGH

Biology is the most powerful technology ever created. DNA is software, proteins are hardware, cells are factories.

Arvind Gupta

Whenever I'm at the gym and the subject of diet comes up, the number one question I'm always asked when people find out that I'm vegan is, "But where do you get your protein?" This is often accompanied by a look of disbelief, or more often, confusion.

Even with the massive explosion in the fake meat market, and the increased awareness of foods such as tofu, tempeh and seitan, a big concern many people have is that if they go vegan or adopt a diet that is more focused on plant-based foods they will not be able to get enough protein in their diet. This is most apparent among men. It must be a throwback to our hunter-gatherer past. Men are often a bit obsessed with protein.

The chances are that if you live in the developed world, whatever diet you're eating, you are not suffering from a protein deficiency. That means you're getting enough protein in your diet to allow the normal functioning of your body. However, there is also a chance that you're not getting enough to support your own personal performance goals. This is especially true if you are on a plant-based diet. In this chapter we're going to go into how much is enough, its sources, and the big differences between plant and animal protein.

WHAT IS PROTEIN?

Protein is an essential nutrient for the human body. It provides the building blocks of muscle, skin, and other tissues, and it plays a vital role in metabolism, cell growth, and hormone production. Proteins are made up of smaller units called amino acids. There are 20 different amino acids that can be used to build proteins, and these amino acids are arranged in a specific order determined by the genetic code.

In general terms, amino acids contribute significantly to the production of protein structures in the body. These are the various types of enzymes that assist the body in digesting food, hormones that communicate information, antibodies that aid in keeping the body's immune system strong as well as playing a crucial role in the production of red blood cells, muscles, and hair. We cannot build critical components in the body if we lack one or more essential amino acids. Since our bodies can only store fats and carbohydrates for future use but not protein, we need to obtain a small amount of each amino acid every day.

WHAT DO THEY DO?

A lot of the amino acids needed in the body can be manufactured by the body, but it needs to get 9 amino acids from the food we eat. There are a wide variety of functions that these amino acids perform:

Valine – The first three on this list, including valine are branched-chain amino acids (often called BCAAs – you might have seen them on the labels of protein powders or pre-workout supplements). Valine plays a vital role in the production of energy and stimulation of muscle growth.

Leucine - Leucine is a critical component of protein synthesis and muscle repair. It also helps regulate blood sugar levels and stimulates wound healing in addition to producing growth hormones.

Isoleucine - Isoleucine has many functions including strengthening your immune system and the production of red blood cells. It also helps regulate energy levels by releasing glucose stored in muscles as well as allowing other processes like muscle metabolism to happen more efficiently.

Lysine - Every cell in your body needs lysine to function at its best. This simple amino acid plays a major role not only in protein synthesis but also absorption of calcium and production of hormones like insulin or epinephrine (adrenaline). It's even necessary when it comes down to creating collagen and elastin - two important structural components in the body.

Methionine - The body needs methionine for metabolism and detoxification. It also helps with tissue growth and absorption of minerals like zinc or selenium, which are crucial for health.

Phenylalanine - Phenylalanine regulates the structure and function of proteins. It is also one of the nutrients your body uses to produce tyrosine, dopamine, epinephrine, and norepinephrine.

Threonine - Without this essential amino acid, your skin may suffer. It's responsible for the structural proteins that hold together cells and provides support in both fat metabolism as well immune function.

Tryptophan - Tryptophan is often associated with drowsiness. It's also the precursor to serotonin, which regulates your appetite, sleep patterns and mood.

Histidine - Histidine is necessary for maintaining the myelin sheath around nerve cells. It is also metabolized into histamine, an important neurotransmitter that helps with immune response, digestion, and sexual function.

The human body is like a puzzle made up of thousands of individual pieces each with its own function, a lot of it made up out of proteins. Throughout our lives, our bodies are continually repaired and replaced with new proteins. To maintain this process (called protein synthesis), amino acids must be continually provided. The breakdown of old body proteins allows some amino acids to be recycled, however, this process isn't perfect, and we therefore need dietary protein to maintain our body's requirement for amino acids.

In children, adolescents, pregnant women, and nursing mothers, adequate protein intake is especially important since it is essential for cell and tissue growth. As well as using proteins to repair and build tissues, your body uses them to regulate metabolic reactions, coordinate bodily functions, maintain a proper pH level, support your immune system, transport and store nutrients, and also provide energy.[1,2] In other words, they do a lot. It's no wonder some people are obsessed with them!

HOW MUCH PROTEIN SHOULD WE EAT EVERY DAY?

This is one of the big questions, and like the other big questions we've come across so far, the boring answer is: *it depends.*

Protein needs vary depending on a number of factors, such as weight, age, the goals of your body composition, and your level of physical activity.

▶ The recommended daily allowance for protein (RDA), as determined by the United States Food and Nutrition Board, is 0.8 grams of protein per kilogram (0.36g/lb) of bodyweight.[3]

According to these recommendations, I need to eat 68g and Aisha almost 49g of protein every day. Based on the number of calories that we both need to eat to maintain energy balance, we can be fairly confident that without any additional supplementation, we would easily be able to reach that figure eating a plant-based diet. For instance, Aisha would just need to eat a little more than 9 cups of boiled spinach. There are certainly more pleasant ways of doing it though (and also potential problems with this approach as we'll see below)!

It's also important to keep in mind that this is the minimum recommended intake most people need to consume each day to maintain muscle growth and repair, meet amino acid requirements, and keep their pH balance in check. In other words, the daily amount you need so that you don't get sick. Protein deficiency results in stunted growth and physical weakness, anemia (not having enough red blood cells), edema (swelling from trapped fluid in the tissues), vascular dysfunction, and impaired immunity.

There is no doubt that increased protein consumption could benefit some people, and in fact will be essential if you are expecting a high level of performance from your body. So again, here it's critical to remember: how much you need depends on what you want to do.

Athletes and very physically active individuals are constantly putting their body under stress, impacting the skeletal muscles, resulting in a greater need for protein than just 0.8g/kg of bodyweight. Greater wear and tear on the body will require a greater source of the material needed for repair.

Endurance athletes need about 1.2-1.4g per kg of bodyweight per day.[4]

If you're looking to use resistance training to build muscle and strength, then you definitely need to up your intake to a minimum of 1g per kg of bodyweight, but some studies recommend even higher – 1.6-1.8g/kg per day.

▶ The International Society of Sports Nutrition goes further and suggests 1.4-2g/kg per day. They endorse this as a quantity that will potentially improve exercise adaptions to training.[5]

That's more than double the amount of protein needed for maintenance. For me it would mean consuming 136g of protein a day (at 1.6g/kg), which is a much harder job than just 68g. In my experience, on a vegan diet, this kind of quantity has needed supplementation in order to get the protein in – but remember, that's only my experience.

If you plan your diet well, it's theoretically possible to do it with whole foods. In practice, it wouldn't be that easy. I'd have to eat 8 ½ cups of beans (almost 1.5kg), or almost 4 ½ cups of tempeh (about 0.75kg) to eat 136g of protein (and that's without taking into account protein quality which we'll cover below). Obviously, you wouldn't rely on just one food source, but beans and soy products are the plant-based foods with the highest protein content. As it's easy to get full when eating them, you might find it hard to reach your target.

There is also some evidence that if you're trying to lose weight by restricting energy intake, but you also want to retain muscle mass, then you need to up the amount of protein even further, to 2.3-3.1g per kg of bodyweight.[6] In bodybuilding terms this is called "cutting." If you already have low body fat, then the higher end of the scale is more appropriate. I know that during my fairly brief time trying out competitive bodybuilding, when I was cutting weight pre-competition, my protein intake was super high – but this was partly because I didn't want to eat too many carbs or fats! On the other hand, when I was "bulking" to put on muscle mass, my protein intake wasn't nearly as high.

The studies are not all in agreement. Some suggest that anything more than 0.8g/kg a day won't do anything, some recommend much higher. When you're calculating your own protein intake, it's worth remembering that it's lean body mass that determines how much protein you need, so you can use that as the basis for working out the value, especially if you're carrying a lot of extra body fat.

Overall, a systematic review and meta-analysis of the effect of protein supplementation found that in healthy adults doing resistance training, ingestion of protein beyond 1.6g/kg of bodyweight per day did not contribute to further gains in fat-free mass. In other words, your body likely cannot process more protein than that and any excess will just be excreted or stored as fat,[7] there's a limit to how much dietary protein can be used for muscle protein synthesis.

RECOMMENDATIONS FOR SPECIAL POPULATIONS

Certain populations may require greater or lesser protein intake for the management of certain medical conditions or to promote growth. The protein needs of pregnant women, nursing mothers, and those with certain health conditions are different to those of the general population

- Protein requirements are higher if you're pregnant or breastfeeding - 0.88-1.1 grams per kilogram of body weight per day.

- Compared to middle-aged adults, older adults may also need more protein - 1.0 to 1.2 grams per kilogram of body weight per day.

- People who suffer from liver or kidney disease are recommended to limit their protein consumption to 0.6 to 0.8 grams of protein per kilogram of body weight per day.

PROTEIN QUALITY

Earlier in the chapter, I said that for Aisha to eat her recommended daily intake of protein, she'd only need to eat 9 cups of cooked spinach. I say "only" but a pile of spinach that large on a plate would be a daunting task to consume, no matter how well seasoned. Quite apart from the effort, this dietary advice has a serious flaw.

We need to get nine essential amino acids from our diet to fulfil our protein needs, and if your food is deficient in even one of the amino acids, it is labeled as an incomplete protein. In reality, all of the amino acids are present in plant-based foods but some of them, including the essential amino acids, may only be present in trace amounts. Spinach, for instance, is considered an incomplete protein. It contains reasonable amounts of lysine, threonine, phenylalanine, isoleucine, valine, and methionine but is low on the other three.

There are some exceptions to the rule, but in general, animal protein is usually complete and plant protein incomplete; the plants that defy this trend include soy, quinoa, and buckwheat.

If you only ate spinach, the issue of complete proteins could be considered a problem. If you only ate one type of food as your main food source, then you'd likely have a lot of other deficiencies as well. In terms of amino acids, if you got your entire daily protein source only from nuts (which would mean an incredibly high fat intake), you would likely not be getting adequate quantities of lysine in your diet. If you got your entire daily protein intake only from vegetable sources (not legumes, beans or anything else), you might have lower than optimal levels of methionine. Both potential diets would be impossible to maintain because it would mean eating no other food whatsoever.

Rice and beans is a combination that is popular in some form on almost every continent, and from the chart you can see why. The relatively low methionine and high lysine content of beans is complimented by the relatively high methionine and low lysine content of rice. It's a combination that has continuously boosted human health throughout its history.

In simple terms, unless you're eating a severely restricted plant-based diet, or one that gets all its calories from nutrient-poor vegan junk food, you're unlikely to be getting an incomplete source of amino acids. Of course, you probably want the quality of your protein intake to be as high as possible, so make sure that your diet is as varied as possible and that your protein comes from a combination of sources. For instance, apart from their low lysine levels, seeds are great source of most of the other essential amino acids and are easy to add to your diet, and soy has a similar amino acid profile to animal protein.

However, completeness is not the only factor that defines a protein's potential quality. The bioavailability and digestibility of plant and animal proteins differ as well.

The Food and Agriculture Organization of the United Nations recommends using the Digestible Indispensable Amino Acid Score (DIASS) to assess protein quality. It's measured by sampling the amino acid content of foods after they have been through the digestive system of a pig – but only as far as the ileum, not all the way out – and accounts for the effects of anti-nutrients (like phytic acid and trypsin inhibitors) on the absorbability of the protein. Pigs are used because of their relative similarity to humans. The samples are evaluated against the amino acid requirements of humans to give a score.

A DIAAS value of over 100 indicates that the protein has extremely high digestibility and is a good complement to proteins of lower quality. Compared to plant-based proteins, animal-based proteins tend to get a higher DIAAS (for instance, whole milk has a score of 114, and pork

117). A score ranging from 75-100 indicates a good protein quality source. Less than 75 indicates a low protein quality source because what is available is likely to be less digestible.

Source	DIASS score	Judged Quality
Wheat	40	Low
Almond	40	Low
Rice	59	Low
Peas	64	Low
Chickpeas	83	High
Soy	90	High
Potato*	100	High

*Although potatoes have a high DIASS, they don't contain a lot of protein by weight, and shouldn't be considered a good source of protein, even though the quality they contain is high.

If your protein requirements are high (for instance if you're doing a lot of endurance or resistance training) and you're relying purely on plant-based protein, then there's a chance that you will need to increase the amount of protein you eat to reach the levels of consumption that you're trying to reach.

A study that looked at competitive endurance athletes determined that vegetarian athletes needed to eat on average an extra 10g of protein to reach their target of 1.2g/kg of bodyweight compared to omnivorous athletes, based on the DIASS of the food they were eating. If they had a target of 1.4g/kg a day, it went up to 22g of protein.[8] Bear in mind that the study wasn't very big (total 75 athletes), and the data retrieved was self-reported, so these figures shouldn't necessarily be considered generalizable rules, but adding an extra protein shake to your daily nutrition might improve your protein uptake if you are on a 100% plant-based diet and have high protein requirements.

PROTEIN-RICH PLANTS

It's totally possible to build muscle mass only eating plants. They contain a lot of protein. Rhinos, gorillas and cows are herbivores and they're huge. Of course, this is a false analogy. Animals have a totally different protein-encoding genetic code to us, and their digestive systems are not the same, but part of the reason for their bulk is the volume of food that they consume. If you eat a lot of plants, you'll end up eating a lot of protein.

If you want to up your intake of plant-based protein, here are the foods you will need to eat:

LEGUMES

These have got to be top of the list both in terms of protein content and all-round health-providing power. Chickpeas (garbanzo beans) are a legume with some of the highest protein quality, even though they don't have the highest protein content. Legume consumption is inversely associated with type 2 diabetes incidence in adults – in a study, those who ate more lentils had the lowest rates of diabetes.[8]

Serving size: *80-90g (½ cup canned)*

Black beans: 8g
Kidney beans: 8g
Lentils: 8g
Peas: 8g
Chickpeas: 7.5g
Pinto beans: 7g

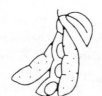

SOY PRODUCTS

Soy is a high-quality protein and is very versatile. You can eat the immature beans, which are called edamame, and they make a great high protein snack. Tempeh is made from the whole fermented beans, so as well as being higher in protein than tofu, it is also higher in a good kind of fiber. Whether you consider tofu, tempeh or soy milk a whole food or not will depend on your personal definition of whole food, and the type of tofu that you eat. A minimally processed block of tofu is very different from one which has been pre-cooked and packaged with flavorings and additives. You can also make tofu yourself from whole soya beans.

Tofu: 20g (*1 cup/248g*)
Tempeh: 31g (*1 cup/166g*)
Edamame beans: 17g (*1 cup/155g*)
Soy milk: 6g (*1 cup/240ml*)

NUTS & SEEDS

Raw, unblanched nuts will have a higher nutritional profile than roasted or blanched ones. They contain many beneficial plant compounds and essential minerals, including iron, calcium, magnesium, selenium and phosphorus. They are also high in fat, so although they are quite a good source of protein, they should be considered a fat source.

Serving size: *28-30g (1oz)*

Hemp seeds: 9.5g
Pumpkin seeds: 8.5g
Almonds: 6g
Flaxseed: 6g
Sunflower seeds: 5.5g
Walnuts: 4.5g
Cashews: 4.5g

CHIA SEEDS

Although these are also a seed, chia gets a section of its own because of its amazing nutrient profile. They contain fiber, omega-3 fatty acids, as well as high levels of iron, calcium, selenium, and magnesium. When they absorb water, they form a gel, which means they can be used in a wide variety of recipes.

1oz (28-30g) – 4.7g

Approx. 10g per tbsp

QUINOA

This grain is unique in that it is a complete protein – it contains all the essential amino acids. It makes a great alternative to rice or couscous as a carbohydrate in a meal, because as well as containing a higher quality protein than other grains, it also contains more protein per gram.

1 cup cooked (200g) – 9g

BUCKWHEAT

This is actually a seed, rather than a grain, high in both protein and fiber. It comes in a variety of formats – flakes, groats (the hulled kernels) and flour. It's used to make soba noodles used in Japanese cooking.

1 cup (170g) – 6g

OATS

Oats are incredibly nutritious, containing a wide variety of important nutrients and vitamins, as well as powerful antioxidants and a high content of beta-glucan, a form of soluble fiber.

1 cup cooked (234g) – 6g

GRAINS

There are other grains that contain good levels of protein – some of which are less commonly available than rice, wheat, oats or barley – but are well worth discovering not just for the potential protein content, but also for their great nutritional value.

Spelt: 11g (*1 cup cooked/194g*)
Teff: 9.8g (*1 cup cooked/252g*)
Freekeh: 10g (*1 cup cooked/200g*)
Amaranth: 9g (*1 cup cooked/246g*)
Millet: 6.1g (*1 cup cooked/174g*)
Brown rice: 5.2g (*1 cup cooked/200g*)

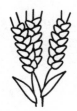

VEGETABLES

Although their protein content is not particularly high, vegetables should be the foundation of a plant-based diet.

Broccoli: 2.6g (*1 cup/90g*)
Asparagus: 2.9g (*1 cup/134g*)
Avocado: 4g (*1 medium avocado*)
Spinach: 5.35g (*1 cup cooked/225g*)

GUAVA

Guava gets a special mention, as the fruit with the highest protein content per gram.

1 cup (165g) – 4.5g

FAKE MEAT

The availability of imitation meat products has created a tipping point in the number of people who are willing to try and eat more plants and less animals. Some companies have worked hard to recreate the meat-eating experience, without the use of animal products, even to the extent that the burgers "bleed" during cooking. Fake meat burgers have become so popular that meat producers are legally trying to prevent the words "beef" or "meat" being used on products made from plants so that they can retain their market share.

While the choice and availability of vegan alternatives means that more people are eating plants, it's important to check the nutritional content of what you're eating. These products will most likely be highly processed, and therefore unsuitable for a whole food diet, unless you make them yourselves from whole food ingredients. Meat analogues are made from a combination of a wide variety of ingredients, from isolated plant proteins like pea or soy, to seitan (made from the wheat protein, gluten), textured vegetable protein, tofu, walnuts or even vegetables themselves. They usually contain vegetable or coconut oil.

Different studies have come up with different results over the contents of imitation burgers when compared to meat burgers. Some have shown that the sodium levels are similar, some that plant-based burgers have a much higher sodium content. In general, protein and saturated fat content is similar in both, but polyunsaturated omega-6 fatty acid content is much higher in the plant-based versions (we'll go into the implications of this in the next chapter). The plant-based burgers also contain more carbohydrates and, significantly, more fiber – beef burgers are fiber free.

Although it potentially can be a useful source of protein, with fake meat, make sure you read the label carefully to see if it fits within your nutritional plan.

CAN YOU HAVE TOO MUCH PROTEIN?

On a 100% plant-based diet, overconsumption of protein alone would be challenging, unless your diet contained a lot of protein powders and isolates. On a whole food plant-based diet, it is almost impossible. You'd most likely suffer from overall overeating and get too full eating the volume of beans and tofu you'd need in order to eat too much protein.

The best answer to the question of how much is too much is – it depends what kind. A lot of the problems associated with protein consumption seem to be associated with eating animal protein, rather than plant protein. Several studies have shown that even as little as a 3% decrease in animal protein in the diet improved mortality outcomes – even after adjusting for the decrease in saturated fat that the reduction would provide. Although cohort studies show that people who eat more protein tend to live shorter lives, this is actually inversely associated with plant protein: people who eat more plant protein live longer.

There are a few reasons why this might be happening. Plant protein in lower in branch chain amino acids (BCAAs) and decreased consumption of BCAAs tends to improve metabolic health. Eating animal protein makes the body produce more IGF-1. IGF-1, insulin-like growth factor, manages the effects of growth hormone in the body, and many studies have flagged it as a risk factor for cancer.[9] Animal products might contain more harmful pollutants – dioxins and PCBs tend to accumulate up the food chain, so they're found in higher concentrations in animals. Whatever the route, reducing animal protein intake can have some very positive health outcomes.

However, even when eating plant protein, there are a couple of things to consider:

Kidney problems: A diet high in protein can be problematic for those with kidney disease, and you should consult a dietitian or general practitioner before increasing the quantities you consume if you have kidney problems.[10]

In general, there is some debate as to whether a high protein diet is safe for kidney health – but the question is again really more concerned with the sources of protein. The hypothesis is that animal proteins are a big source of sulfur-containing amino acids which increases acidity in the body leading to excess pressure on the kidneys.

On the contrary, there is some evidence that protein specifically from plant-based sources may be beneficial for lowering the risk of kidney disease. Using data from the National Health and Nutrition Examination Survey III, researchers examined the health data of 1,065 people with chronic kidney disease. Plant protein consumption was found to lower the risk of death for people with chronic kidney disease when animal was replaced by plant protein.[11]

Weight Gain: Like carbohydrates and fats, excess protein consumption can also lead to weight gain because eating more protein than your body needs can mean excess energy is stored as fat. When you eat too many calories and increase your protein intake at the same time, this may result in weight gain over time.[12]

SOY: GOOD OR BAD?

The final topic I want to cover in this chapter is the sometimes-controversial subject of soy. As we covered above, soy is an excellent source of protein. It is one of the plant-based sources with the highest quality, and is a great way of adding diversity to a vegan or vegetarian diet because of the different forms it comes in. It has also been linked to a number of health benefits, including protecting heart health, managing blood sugar levels, and reducing cancer risk.

However, there are some very loud anti-soy voices that might cause you to question whether it is a good idea to make soy a large part of your diet, or for it even feature at all. The main issue revolves around soy's high content of isoflavones, a kind of polyphenol that are often called phytoestrogens. Although they differ from estrogen in many ways, some believe that they can mimic estrogen in the body, causing a host of problems because they disrupt the endocrine system. Men are often concerned that eating too much soy will have a feminizing effect, however a meta-analysis showed that soy consumption didn't have an impact on bioavailable testosterone levels.[13] Some opponents to soy also claim that consumption can lead to thyroid problems, which has been seen in animals, but not in humans with healthy thyroid function.[14]

One thing that is of concern is that most of the soybeans grown worldwide are genetically modified (GMO). Often the plants are engineered to be resistant to herbicides, which means that they can be treated with chemicals like glyphosate. Although the Environmental Protection Agency in the US has issued a statement to the effect that glyphosate does not pose a risk to human health, there is some controversy over its use and the potential increased risk of cancer, endocrine disruption, celiac disease, and autism that consuming it might incur.[15]

WHEN ENOUGH IS ENOUGH

Have we become a bit obsessed with protein as a culture? Probably a little bit. But that doesn't mean it's not important. If you're fairly sedentary you will have low calorie and protein requirements. You will very likely get everything you need from eating a varied diet without thinking too much about it.

But if you are engaged in training of any sort or trying to change your body composition, then it really is something you need to pay attention to. Work out how much you are getting on a daily basis and try and get some idea of the quality of the protein as well. Bear in mind that you might need to increase your intake if the quality is consistently on the lower end of the scale. Remember, beyond a certain point your body might not be able to process excess protein, and also remember that diet creates changes over the long term, not just in one single meal.

On a WFPB diet, protein will always come packaged with some carbohydrate – this is how plant protein exists in the natural world – so the difficulty will always be maintaining the correct energy balance while getting the amount you need. The macronutrient that can have a huge impact on energy balance is fat, which we are going to look at in the next chapter.

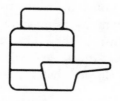

CHAPTER 7

FAT-FREE IS NOT THE ANSWER

Two forms of fat that are vitally important for brain health are cholesterol and saturated fat.

David Perlmutter

Fat is a controversial subject. Long seen as the enemy when it comes to weight loss and heart health, it's also well known that not all fats are created equal. Some fats are essential for good health, some are best avoided. Research on the subject is evolving, and there are powerful industries involved that have a personal stake in keeping some fats on the table.

The key is to choose the right types of fats and to consume them in moderation. This means that we must try to understand what the "right types" are!

Besides providing energy, some fats are classed as essential nutrients. The wrong type of fat or too much fat can, however, negatively impact our health. Furthermore, fats make what we eat more interesting, contributing to the specific texture, appearance, and flavor of food.

From a performance perspective, one of the main questions to ask yourself is whether you want to try and change your source of fuel, and we'll discuss that at the end of the chapter. Before then, we'll look more generally at the health outcomes that are affected by fat consumption as this will affect long term performance, in particular cardiovascular health.

Fat is a tricky subject. No one doubts its importance for human health, but there is a lot of disagreement as to what constitutes a healthy source. A very low fat or fully fat-free diet is definitely not the answer.

Although it comes from a very small study, research found a link between low-fat diets and lowered testosterone levels,[1] and among other things testosterone plays a key role in muscle adaption to training for both men and women.

WHAT ARE FATS?

The fats you find in vegetable oils and the fat that might find in the adipose tissue around your waistline are made of the same components – triglycerides. Often the term fat is used to refer to all lipids, which include waxes, sterols (like cholesterol), free fatty acids, and phospho-lipids (the key component in cell membranes). They are composed of carbon, oxygen and hydrogen and are insoluble in water.

Besides supplying energy to the body, dietary fats also play an important role in a variety of bodily functions. Our bodies need fats to maintain the structural integrity of their cells and membranes, for instance, around 60 percent of our brain is fat. They are also needed to store fat-soluble vitamins A, D, E, and K. Chemical compounds of fat play crucial roles in the development of the nervous system and in inflammatory responses. By storing fat, the body guarantees a future energy source, protects vital organs, and provides insulation.

HOW MUCH SHOULD YOU HAVE?

Usually, when I'm working with a client who is trying a plant-based diet, I don't pay too much attention to fat. That's not to say that I don't think it's important, but that it often takes care of itself.

The dietary guidelines state that you should get 20-35% of daily calories from fats. For Aisha, eating 2,232 calories a day, that would be 446-781 calories or about 50-87g. She could eat a 200g bag of cashew nuts (about 1.3 cups) and that would be the upper limit of daily fat that she should eat, but she would still need to eat over 1,000 calories or else be in a significant calorie deficit that day and likely be very hungry.

If you have a bad junk food habit and are regularly ordering delivery vegan burgers and fries on several nights a week, or if you survive solely on potato chips, nuts or other high fat snacks then by all means take a moment to calculate the fat content of what you're consuming and see how far it fits within the recommendations. It's well worth looking at the nutritional information for the processed food that you regularly like to eat (if you do eat any), to give yourself an idea of how far you're sticking to your nutrition goals. Usually, its these kinds of foods that will blow up a nutrition plan.

If you're eating a plant-based diet, and you're not relying heavily on fried foods or nuts, it's quite hard to eat more than the top end of 35% of your daily calories from fat as long as you're not overconsuming calories. If you're going strictly whole food, it's almost impossible – unless you go really heavy on the nuts. Remember, from a macronutrient point of view, I tend to consider nuts to be a source of fat, rather than protein, even though they do contain a reasonable amount of protein.

If you're trying to lose weight, concentrating on the fat content of food will be less beneficial than paying attention to the total amount of calories consumed and making sure your protein intake is sufficient. Once you have the right calorie balance, and you've got a good level of protein intake, you'll find you will probably be absolutely fine for fat. The one thing that I try and make my clients more aware of is to understand the sources of the fat they consume. However, with some clients I do focus on fat. If they have specific goals for body composition, like reducing body fat below 12%, then it takes a different kind of planning.

Different types of fat exist - some of which are considered harmful, some of which are considered healthy. Unsaturated fats, such as mono-unsaturated and polyunsaturated fat, are considered healthier than saturated and trans fats. Let's go over each of them in detail.

CHOLESTEROL

At the heart of the story of fat is cholesterol, a fatty, waxy substances that circulates in our blood. It is essential for making hormones and for maintaining healthy cells membranes and it is produced by the liver. As cholesterol doesn't dissolve in water, the liver produces lipoproteins so that it can be carried in the bloodstream, and these lipoproteins come in two different densities, high and low. This gives the distinction between the types of cholesterol found in the body:

◇ **LDL cholesterol** is carried by low-density lipoproteins – too much is unhealthy and causes clogs in the arteries, it's often called "bad cholesterol."

◇ **HDL cholesterol** is carried by high-density lipoprotein – it can help to clear your arteries of excess LDL cholesterol.

If you have too much LDL cholesterol in the body, it can build up in the walls of the arteries to form plaques which narrow the blood vessel, reducing blood flow and increasing the chances of blood clots which might lead to heart attack or stroke.

The research is mixed as to whether dietary cholesterol increases levels of LDL cholesterol in the blood, although recent findings suggest that there are some links. One study which analyzed 30,000 people over a period of almost 18 years found that increased cholesterol consumption, in particular from eggs, resulted in an increased risk of cardiovascular disease.[2] If you're following an exclusively plant-based diet, this question is essentially irrelevant as cholesterol is only found in animal products.

SATURATED FATS

Saturated fats are highly concentrated with hydrogen atoms – none of the carbon atoms have double bonds with other carbon atoms, they are all bonded to hydrogen. They are found in the highest quantities in animal products such as red meat, poultry, and dairy products, but they are also present in plants. Oils that are solid at room temperatures, such as palm oil, palm kernel oil, and coconut oil contain saturated fat. Therefore, baked goods – even vegan ones – can easily contain a high percentage of saturated fats if they are made with these oils or vegan butter, which is often made from them.

For many years, saturated fat has been at the center of the fight against coronary heart disease. Together with cholesterol, it has long been considered the primary contributor to this health epidemic. Current recommendations concentrate on the idea that replacing saturated with polyunsaturated fat lowers the risk of heart disease, as higher intakes of saturated fat are associated with higher levels of the bad kind of cholesterol in the blood stream and higher incidence of cardiovascular disease.[3]

However, the research is also dotted with studies which refute this association, or claim that it is not causal, that high cholesterol levels can be caused by many other factors. Not all of these studies are highly regarded by the scientific community. Even so, the idea that replacing saturated fat with an intake of increased polyunsaturated fat will only lead to positive outcomes is also questionable. When you start to consider the sources of the polyunsaturated fats, as we will see below, you will begin to understand why.

▶ The American Heart Association (AHA) recommends that no more than 5-6% of daily calories should come from saturated fat.[4]

For example, Aisha, eating 2,232 calories a day, would only be able to eat up to 156 calories from saturated fat, which is equivalent to 17g. In real food terms, that's 4 avocados or less than 1 cup of Brazil nuts.

In general, plant-based diets are low in saturated fat, especially if the concentration is on whole food sources.

TRANS FAT

Trans fat is less ambiguous. It is a type of fat that has been chemically altered to be more solid at room temperature. This process, known as hydrogenation, increases the shelf life of food products made with trans fats. If you look on food packaging, you might see them labelled as "partially hydrogenated oils." Often fast-food restaurants will use trans fats for frying as they can be reused multiple times in commercial fryers.

Use of trans fats in food production began to be increasingly popular after the 1950s, as processed foods became more and more widespread, until the links were discovered between consumption and bad health outcomes. Now everyone knows trans fats are no good, although you might still find them in some processed foods. Eating them can increase levels of the bad LDL cholesterol in the blood and reduce levels of good HDL cholesterol. Again, this increase in bad cholesterol can lead to a higher risk of heart disease and other health problems.

Some trans fats are naturally occurring in dairy and meat, but the vast majority are created through the hydrogenation process, and it is unclear whether naturally occurring trans fats have the same effects as artificial. It depends on who is doing the research – the meat industry is keen not to have the bad association of trans fat. A recent meta-analysis determined that regardless of the source, natural or industrially pro-duced, trans fats have the same effect on cholesterol – increasing LDL and decreasing HDL.[5] Another reason to avoid eating animal products – a rib-eye steak can contain more than 4g of trans fat.

▶ There is no recommended level of daily intake because there is no safe level of consumption for trans fats.

They have been banned in the United States since 2018. Still, it is important to check food labels carefully to avoid products that contain high levels of trans fat – before 2006 it was impossible to know whether products even contained trans fats in the US, as it was not mandatory to list it on the Nutrition Facts panel on the packaging. Now trace amounts in food are still allowed. Many convenience foods might still contain them, such as frozen pizzas and fried foods, but you also find them in margarine, cookies, and cakes (especially the frosting). If you're eating a plant-based whole food diet, you should never encounter them at all.

MONOUNSATURATED FATS

The name monounsaturated comes from the fact that these types of fats have only a single carbon double bond in the molecule: they are not saturated with hydrogen atoms. They are liquid at room temperature. For example, canola, peanut, and olive oils contain monounsaturated fats. They are also present in olives and avocados, and of all the nuts, almonds have the highest content.

Several studies have indicated that monounsaturated fats may protect the heart, although the consensus is not to recommend them as an intervention for preventing cardiovascular disease.[6] There is also some evidence that they may improve cholesterol and insulin levels, as well as help manage blood sugar control.

POLYUNSATURATED FATS

Polyunsaturated fat molecules contain more than one carbon double bond. At room temperature, they are liquid. Soybean oil, safflower oil, corn oil, sunflower oil, walnuts, and flaxseeds are predominant sources of polyunsaturated fat. For those not following a plant-based diet, they're typically found in fatty fish, such as salmon, tuna, herring, mackerel, and trout.

As we said above, most public health recommendations endorse the idea that an increase in polyunsaturated fat and a decrease in saturated fat intake can reduce the risk of cardiovascular disease by lowering levels of LDL cholesterol blood. However, there is also some evidence that polyunsaturated fats induce benefits to the cardiovascular system, due to their effects on the heart, vasculature, and blood.[7]

Just like amino acids, there are some fatty acids that the body cannot produce itself. These are called essential fatty acids of which there are two groups: omega-6 and omega-3 fatty acids. These will be discussed in depth later in the chapter, as well as in Chapter 8.

THE WHOLE FOOD HYPOTHESIS: THERE IS NO SUCH THING AS A HEALTHY FAT

Depending on how strict your interpretation of a whole food diet is, it is highly likely that oils of any sort are off the table. Most vegetable oils are highly processed, and even if they're cold-pressed, they are still not whole foods. One single nutrient has been isolated and extracted from the package of nutrients that the whole food contains.

The whole food community believes – possible quite correctly – that we've been conditioned by the multi-billion-dollar cooking oil industry into believing that some fats are healthy. The reward systems in our brain are pre-programmed to crave fat-rich foods (just like they respond to sugar-rich foods), and the effects can be disastrous for our health. If you think about the Dr Fuhrman's "health" equation, oil has a high calorie and a low nutrient content, which results in a low health outcome.

From the perspective of cardiovascular health, a single meal high in fat can impair artery function for hours after consumption. Fat has an impact on the functioning of endothelial cells, the lining of arteries which controls their relaxation and contraction.[8] Not only is there an increase in serum triglyceride levels, but there's a higher likelihood of the formation of foam cells, the precursors to arterial plaques which cause atherosclerosis.[9] Of course, this impact isn't permanent, but if you're regularly eating high-fat meals, you'll spend longer in a postprandial state where your arteries' function has been compromised. And this kind of impact is most noticeable when animal products are consumed – for instance, the same impairment of arterial function wasn't found when whole nuts were the source of fats.[10]

So, if you're strictly following a whole food plant-based diet, that means to get enough dietary fat, you need to eat olives rather than olive oil, coconuts rather than coconut oil, flaxseed rather than flaxseed oil and so on. You might find getting enough fat in your diet can actually be quite challenging. This is another case where I make sure my clients are calculating how much fat they are eating - too little can cause problems with recovery, especially if there are engaged in high intensity training. On a whole food diet, you definitely need nuts!

Even if your interpretation of a whole food diet allows you to consume vegetable oils in some format, it may be worthwhile limiting your consumption and looking to find your dietary fats from other sources as it turns out that vegetable oils might not be that great for a number of reasons.

THE PROBLEMS WITH VEGETABLE OIL

The edible oils that are extracted from plants are usually called vegetable oils, although most of them come from seeds or nuts.

In many vegetable oils, the predominant fatty acid is linoleic acid, which is a polyunsaturated omega-6 fatty acid. For instance, you find it in large quantities in corn, sunflower, canola and soybean oil. The consumption of omega-6 fatty acids is necessary for survival as they cannot be manufactured by the body, and they play a significant role in brain function and are crucial for growth and development. However, there is some question over the effects of consuming them in excess.

Specifically, the problem seems to be with the balance of omega-6 versus omega-3 fatty acids in the diet: consuming too much omega-6 and not enough omega-3 can provoke an inflammatory response in the body. This can significantly increase the risk of chronic inflammatory diseases such as cardiovascular disease, obesity, and Alzheimer's disease, among others.[11,12] The AHA is keen to stress that consumption of omega-6 fatty acids is not pro-inflammatory on its own – hence the official recommendations to replace saturated fats with polyunsaturated ones for improved heart health.[13] Yet, even with these recommendations, incidences of chronic inflammatory diseases are increasing. It's very possible that part of the reason is the imbalance in the essential fatty acids in modern diets. Ancestral ratios of omega-3 to omega-6 were roughly 1:1, but now, with the increase in consumption of highly processed seed oils, it can be as high as 1:20. We're getting way too much omega-6.

Here's a simplification of the science behind the problems with the imbalance. Both types of essential fatty acids are precursors to signaling molecules (called eicosanoids) which help regulate inflammation in the body, and the same enzymes are used in the pathways to create them from both types of fatty acids. This means they are essentially competing for the conversion enzymes, and a huge imbalance in the ratio will mean fewer anti-inflammatory molecules are created from omega-3 fatty acids, even if they are present in the diet. The positive effects of consuming omega-3 fatty acids have been well documented, and we will look into them in the next chapter.

COOKING WITH VEGETABLE OILS

Humans have been cooking with oil for millennia. The Ancient Egyptians used palm oil; the Ancient Greeks used olive oil. When oil is heated it breaks down in a complex process of chemical degradation. Part of that process means that in the presence of air and water the fatty acids in the oil oxidize. For modern consumers, it means that to keep the oils stable so that they have a longer shelf life, manufacturers add preservatives. A controversial one called tertiary butylhydroquinone (TBHQ) is often used. It acts as an antioxidant but ingesting high levels has been linked to a number of a number of health problems in both animals and humans.

Unlike palm and olive oil, which were traditionally produced by pressing the fruits to squeeze out the oil, much of the cooking oil that is available on the market today is produced using high heat, solvents, and bleaching agents.

During cooking, when fatty acids oxidize, they produce aldehydes, ketones and alcohols. Part of the delicious flavor of fried food is down to these compounds. However, in high quantities aldehydes can be potentially damaging to human health – in exceedingly high doses, some can even be lethal. Don't worry though, the amounts you could produce in any kind of kitchen would never reach those levels, and in general, the production of harmful aldehydes is less of an issue when you cook at home – research has not shown that the quantities involved will have an impact on human health. The problem is significantly increased when oil is reheated multiple times, as can happen in fast food restaurants that produce a lot of fried food.

Fatty acids which are more unsaturated tend to oxidize more quickly than those which are more saturated – in other words, poly-unsaturated fats degrade the fastest when exposed to heat. All oils have a smoke point – the temperature at which the oil will start to smoke – and it's important not to heat the oil above its smoke point as this also drastically increases oxidation. For instance, sunflower oil has a lower smoke point than olive oil, so the latter makes a better choice for the high temperatures involved in cooking.

Another problem with heating oil is that it can increase its content of trans fatty acids. We've already rung the warning bell for consuming trans fats: there's really nothing positive about them. Avoid them in order to maintain optimal health and long-term performance. Surprisingly, vegetable oils which have not been hydrogenated can also contain trans fats. One study looked at canola and soybean oil that was purchased in the United States and determined that the trans-fat content of the oil was 0.56% and 4.2% of the total fatty acids respectively.[14] Another study – this one looking at soybean oil, groundnut oil, olive oil and rapeseed oil in India – found that heating the oils increased their content of trans fats by up to 5%.[15]

In the USA, food can be labelled as containing no trans fat if it contains less then 0.5g of trans fat per serving. So it's highly likely that the oil you buy in the supermarket may contain trans fats, and more if you cook with it.

COOKING WITHOUT OIL

If you decide to follow a whole food diet that cuts out oil, you are faced with the dilemma of how to cook without using it. It's not too complicated but requires a bit of pre-planning to make sure you have the right ingredients and equipment. Here are the ways to approach it with different cooking methods:

Stir-frying (or sautéing): this is technically the most challenging but requires the least extra things. Use a small amount of water or broth, adding only a little at a time (1-2 tbsp) so that the food doesn't stick. Don't add too much otherwise the food in the bottom of the pan will boil, and the rest will steam, but add as much as you need to keep it from burning.

Roasting: you'll need to use parchment paper on your baking sheets or roasting trays, but then you can just add the vegetables you want. They'll cook well without the oil, and they won't stick to the pan. Make sure you season them well – you can use a little liquid (broth or sauce) as a seasoning.

Baking: replace the oil with applesauce or mashed banana. This might make whatever you are baking quite a bit sweeter, but fruit purées will help create the same consistency as using oil or butter.

Deep-frying: there's not really an alternative to this! Make baked potatoes rather than fries is the best advice! You can look for recipes which coat the ingredients in a crispy baked crust if you're looking for the same crunch you get from deep fried food.

THE KETOGENIC DIET

You've probably come across the ketogenic diet at some point. It is at the opposite end of the spectrum to a whole food diet because fat figures heavily. It is the most extreme end of a low carbohydrate approach, where fat is used as the main source of calories, with a moderate amount of protein.

The diet was originally developed as a treatment for epilepsy but has become wildly popular due to the numerous health benefits it appears to confer. It can lower abdominal fat levels, lower blood sugar and insulin levels, lower triglycerides in the blood and increase levels of good HDL cholesterol.[16] Some of this might sound counterintuitive for a diet that is high in fat.

By dramatically restricting carbs, it forces the body to use fat as a fuel source. When intake is reduced to less than 50g a day (5-10% of daily calories), you induce a state called ketosis in your body. Rather than using glucose to produce energy, the breakdown of fat in the liver produces ketone bodies which are used instead.

The diet is particularly beneficial for those who are suffering from metabolic syndrome or have the symptoms of insulin resistance – in other words, if a big change needs to be made to your lifestyle to improve your baseline health. From the perspective of athletic performance, more research is needed as to whether a keto diet would be beneficial. Current research suggests that the diet is more suitable for endurance athletes to enhance performance compared to those that require short bursts of energy, although the results are ultimately inconclusive as to whether measurable outcomes, like changes to VO2 max would be improved.[17] If you do decide to try changing to a ketogenic diet, you will need to allow your body to adapt long-term to the diet to get the best performance out of it.

CAN YOU GO PLANT-BASED KETO?

The simple answer is yes, but not on a whole food diet. Whole food keto isn't possible even if you eat animal products. It's very hard to get enough fat on a whole food diet that isn't either packaged with carbohydrate or protein.

Plant-based diets and ketogenic diets both have well-established health benefits – and benefits in similar domains – for instance, they both reduce the risk of chronic diseases like type 2 diabetes and cardio-vascular disease. However, there's no evidence that these benefits would be compounded by following a vegan ketogenic diet, or how they'd interact, as no research has been done yet.

The hardest part of a vegan keto diet is not to go over your limit of carbohydrates as most plant-based foods are high in carbohydrates. To that end you will probably feel that your diet is severely restricted. You will need to avoid grains, starchy vegetables and legumes, which normally form the backbone of a plant-based diet. Instead focus on coconut products (the cream, milk, flesh and oil), nuts and seeds (and nut butters), leafy greens and other non-starchy vegetables, soy products (tofu and tempeh), avocados and berries. And of course, oil itself!

Adding vegetable oils, especially olive oil, to your meals is an effective way of getting enough calories in and hitting the required fat macro percentages for the diet.

Remember that in a ketogenic diet, you will need to keep track of how much protein you're eating. The recommendations are that you only consume 10-20% of your daily calories from protein sources. If you eat too much protein, your body might not enter a state of ketosis and gluconeogenesis might occur instead. This also takes place in the liver, where amino acids (from protein), glycerol (from fat) and lactate and pyruvate (compounds that occur in the process of glucose metabolism) are used to make glucose which is used as the energy source. This is more likely to happen on an omnivorous diet, as carb free protein sources are more readily available.

If you're serious about going plant-based keto, you will also need to make sure your diet is adequately supplemented. Because it will be so restricted, it could easily end up lacking in essential micronutrients. This is the topic we are going to cover in depth in the next chapter.

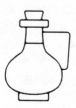

CHAPTER 8

WHAT'S MISSING?

No evidence compels the conclusion that the minimum required intake of any vitamin comes close to the optimum intake that sustains good health.

Linus Pauling

Micronutrients are essential nutrients that are required in small amounts for proper growth and development. Although they are needed in very small quantities, they are essential for a number of important biochemical processes, including enzyme function, cell division, and DNA synthesis. Without adequate levels of micronutrients, these processes cannot occur properly, leading to poor health and stunted growth.

Although plant foods provide many essential nutrients, there are a few that are difficult or impossible to obtain. To maintain health and to ensure you can reach your maximum performance potential, we must be aware of these substances and supplement our diets if necessary.

This is a long chapter. There's a lot to cover - we are going to discuss which nutrients you may be missing while eating a plant-based diet and solutions to how you can make up for potential deficiencies.

WHAT IS A NUTRIENT DEFICIENCY?

The body suffers from nutritional deficiencies if it does not receive enough vitamins or minerals. Many health problems may be caused by nutrient deficiencies, such as stunted growth and hair loss, and some deficiencies can even lead to serious medical conditions, such as dementia.

Extreme nutrient deficiencies are at the far end of the scale. But it is a scale that doesn't necessarily have a clear limit at the other end. It is important to consider how much of a micronutrient you need to perform at your best.

According to World Health Organization, around 80 percent of people in the world suffer from iron deficiency, the most common nutritional deficiency.[1] If severe iron deficiency is present, it can result in anemia, which can interfere with cardiac health, cause pregnancy complications such as premature births, and can delay the development and growth of children. Also common are calcium and vitamin D imbalances, as well as sub-optimal levels of B12.

These are figures for omnivores. When you start restricting your diet, it can get worse. If your plant-based diet isn't planned carefully, it may be missing certain essential nutrients. Let's go over each of them and see how you can make sure you get enough of them in your diet.

VITAMIN B12

This is the main one. Theoretically, everything else, all the other essential vitamins and minerals, can be supplied by a whole food plant-based diet and regular exposure to the sun. In reality, modern vegan diets contain a lot of foods which have been fortified with B12, so you're likely to get some from your diet anyway.

Vitamin B12 is a critical nutrient that is necessary for cellular division, to replicate and repair DNA, for metabolic processes like making fatty and amino acids and maintaining the health of the nervous and cardiovascular system. It's used by every cell in the body. Research suggests that vegans are frequently deficient in the vitamin.[2] Even if you don't have a deficiency, levels might not be high enough for best performance, especially over the long term. In fact, research also shows that even a third of non-vegetarians are not getting enough for optimal health, and this figure increases to 50% in women, and 60% in pregnant women. For plant-based eaters it is more than 85% and if you've been vegan for more than 10 years, then it is all the way up to 100%.[3]

When the body does not have adequate amounts of vitamin B12, it cannot break down homocysteine, an amino acid linked to fatigue, weakness, and numbness. Raised levels of homocysteine in the blood have also been linked to an increased risk of dementia – in particular Alzheimer's disease.[4] Likewise, low levels of B12 are associated with higher levels of methylmalonic acid in the blood, which can be an indicator of kidney disease or renal failure.

The liver can store vitamin B12, which means it may take years before low B12 intake results in a full-blown deficiency.[5] A doctor may consider your B12 levels to be "normal," but they may not be optimal. Maintaining optimal levels of B12 and low serum homocysteine is imperative if you eat a plant-based diet, especially if you have been doing so for many years.

VITAMIN B12 SOURCES

Since B12 cannot be manufactured by the body, it must be consumed in the diet. Proteins are bound to vitamin B12, and it is found in all animal products, including milk, eggs, fish, meat, and poultry – it's only not found in honey.

People who eat plant-based diets need to supplement their daily nutritional needs with fortified foods.

Plant-Based Sources of Vitamin B12

Food	Amount	B12 (mcg)
Rice drink	8 oz	1.5
Nutritional yeast	1 tbsp	4.0
Protein bar (fortified)	1	1.0 – 2.0
Cereals (fortified)	½ cup	<1.0 – 6.1
Soy milk (fortified)	8 oz	<1.0 – 3.0
Meat analogues	1 serving	1.2 – 4.2

Many foods are fortified with B12 vitamin, such as breakfast cereals, fake meat, soy milk, and nutritional yeast. It is possible to fortify them anywhere from a small amount to 200% of the RDA. Because these products may not all be fortified, and fortification can evolve over time, you should always carefully read the ingredients list and the nutritional panel of products.

To improve the absorbability of the vitamin, space out the time when you consume the fortified foods – in other words, don't leave it all to just one meal a day. In order to reach the recommended amounts of B12 in your diet, you will need to consume fortified products in different quantities, depending on which ones you eat. For many this is just not feasible, and you might find a B12 supplement to be more efficient.

HOW MUCH B12 DO YOU NEED?

This is a more complicated question than it might appear. On average – if you're gastrointestinal tract is functioning normally – an adult loses approximately 1 mcg of B12 a day. To accommodate for that, the recommended dietary allowances from the Institute of Medicine are as follows:

Recommended Dietary Allowances (RDAs) for Vitamin B12

Age	Male	Female	Pregnancy	Breastfeeding
0–6 months	0.4 mcg	0.4 mcg		
7–12 months	0.5 mcg	0.5 mcg		
1–3 years	0.9 mcg	0.9 mcg		
4–8 years	1.2 mcg	1.2 mcg		
9–13 years	1.8 mcg	1.8 mcg		
14+ years	2.4 mcg	2.4 mcg	2.6 mcg	2.8 mcg

The recommended intake for adults is more than twice the amount that is lost per day because of poor absorption – and absorption is worse when the vitamin is taken in supplement form. One study found that up to 10 mcg is needed in oral supplementation to replace the 1 mcg lost a day.[6] However, another determined that even supplementing with 10 mcg a day failed to bring homocysteine down to optimal levels in the body, suggesting that even higher doses are needed for optimal health.[7]

Part of the problem might be that the current RDA is based on a study from the 1950s which looked only a blood counts – it could be that replacing 1 mcg a day is enough to maintain adequate blood cell production, but more is needed to make sure the body can perform at its best. How much? As always, it depends. What you're eating and doing will always make a big difference. It is worth noting that in a randomized controlled trial, vegetarians and vegans with a marginal deficiency were found to have adequate blood serum levels of vitamin B12 after taking a 50 mcg a day supplement.[8]

A NOTE ON B12 SUPPLEMENTATION

Many people would benefit from B12 supplementation, even omnivores. It's better to take a specific B12 supplement, rather than a multivitamin if you have decided to supplement, so that you can make sure that you're getting an adequate amount of the vitamin.

Typically, B12 supplements contain cyanocobalamin, a form the body converts quickly into the co-enzymes, methylcobalamin and adenosylcobalamin. Cyanocobalamin contains a molecule of cyanide, which has sometimes put off alternative health practitioners from recommending its use as a supplement, but the amount of cyanide in a supplement is way less than the amount consumed on a daily basis from other sources and is considered to have no physiological effect. The most stable form of the vitamin is cyanocobalamin, which has been widely studied.[9] Due to its ability to prevent and reverse deficiency, it is frequently recommended by healthcare professionals.

The Institute of Medicine (IOM) in the United States bases its RDAs (in the table above) on the amount of B12 needed to treat pernicious anemia (a deficiency in the production of red blood cells). The European Food Safety Authority (EFSA) takes a slightly different approach and bases its recommendations on the amount of B12 supplementation needed to maintain suitable levels of certain bio-markers (serum B12, homocysteine and methylmalonic acid), so its adequate intake levels are higher than the IOM's RDAs.

All of that will go some way to explaining why the following chart has such a wide range of recommendations for supplementation. You can stick with the lower end from the IOM, or the upper end from the EFSA. The figures are calculated on the absorbability of cyanocobalamin. You can choose to supplement within a wide range of frequency, from several times a day to just once a week.

Cyancobalamin recommendations for vegans to meet IOM's RDA & EFAS's AI[10] (IOM-EFSA)

Age	3x day µg	2x day µg	1x day µg	3x week µg	2x week µg	1x week µg
6 months	0.2	0.2	0.4			
7-11 months	0.2-0.5	0.3-1.0	0.5-10			
1-3 years	0.3-0.5	0.5-1.0	0.9-10			
4-6 years	0.4-0.5	0.6-1.0	1.4-10	100-500	500-1000	1000-2500
7-8 years	0.4-0.7	0.6-1.4	1.5-50	100-500	500-1000	1000-2500
9-10 years	0.5-0.8	0.8-1.8	2-50	250-500	500-1000	1000-2500
11-13 years	0.6-1.0	0.9-2	5-50	250-500	500-1000	1000-2500
14 years	0.8-1.2	1.2-5	5-100	250-1000	500-1000	1250-2500
>15 years	0.8-1.3	1.2-5	5-100	250-1000	500-1250	1250-2500
Pregnant	0.9-1.5	1.3-5	10-250			
Breastfeeding	1.0-1.7	1.4-5	10-250			

There doesn't appear to be a definite point at which supplementing with B12 becomes unsafe – there's no Tolerable Upper Intake Level as it is non-toxic. However, if you have kidney disease (and 38% of Americans over the age of 65 have chronic kidney disease), you should speak to your doctor about how to supplement B12 appropriately.

OMEGA-3 FATTY ACIDS

Omega-3 fatty acids are polyunsaturated fats that have a variety of health benefits. As we touched on in Chapter 7, these essential fatty acids play an integral role in supporting cardiovascular, brain, kidney and overall cellular health, as well as reducing inflammation and promoting healthy skin and eyes. The three major types of omega-3 fats are alpha-linolenic acid (ALA), eicosapentaenoic acid (EPA), and docosahexaenoic acid (DHA). Algae and plants contain ALA, while fish like salmon and tuna contain EPA and DHA.

Of the three, only ALA is found in most of the plants we eat, and as it is not synthesized by our bodies, we must obtain it through our diets. EPA and DHA can also be found in some kinds of algae, which is why fish, who eat the algae are a good source of these fatty acids. ALA can also be converted by our body into the other long-chain omega-3s, EPA and DHA. However, the conversion is highly inefficient and only about 7-15% of the ALA is converted into EPA and DHA. As a result, levels of these two omega-3 fatty acids are 30% lower in vegetarians and 50% lower in vegans, compared to omnivores. However, currently there is insufficient evidence to determine whether this will lead to negative health outcomes.[11]

An adult male should consume 1,600 milligrams of ALA per day, and an adult female should consume 1,100 milligrams per day. This amount increases for women who are pregnant or breastfeeding (1,400 mg & 1,300 mg respectively), or for those with a reduced ability to convert ALA, like the elderly. For good conversion levels of ALA to EPA and DHA, research recommends taking in at least 2,000 milligrams of ALA per day.[12]

Remember, as we discussed in the previous chapter, getting the right balance of omega-3 to omega-6 fatty acids is important. So, if your diet is high in polyunsaturated fatty acids from vegetable oils, make sure you are eating good sources of food which contain plenty of ALA. If you're not on a whole food diet, adding flax seed oil to smoothies works really well.

Plant-based sources of alpha-linolenic acid (ALA)

Food	Serving Size	ALA content (mg)
Pumpkin seeds	1 oz	31
Brussels sprouts	½ cup	80
Cauliflower	½ cup	104
Wheat germ	1 oz	108
Tofu, firm	½ cup	733
Soybeans, cooked	½ cup	820
Soy oil	1 oz	933
Canola oil	1 oz	1279
Hemp Seeds	1 oz	1567
Walnuts	1 oz	2570
Chia seeds	1 oz	4596
Flaxseed	1 oz	4614
Flaxseed oil	1 tbsp	7258

A NOTE ON OMEGA 3 SUPPLEMENTS

Currently, researchers do not have a clear understanding of how much DHA or EPA to take as supplements. There is not a great deal of certainty when it comes to the optimal dosage as it varies significantly from individual to individual, so you should always consult your physician before commencing any regime of supplementation. A general recommendation is to consume 200-300 mg of DHA each day.[13] Obviously, if you're following a plant-based diet, you'll need to get your supplements from an algal source, rather than fish oil, and this will come with its own additional benefits. Due to ocean pollution, fish may contain a variety of things which are dangerous to human health, like dioxins, PCBs and heavy metals.

VITAMIN D

Just like vitamin B12, this isn't necessarily a problem only for people who follow a plant-based diet. Many people have sub-optimal levels of vitamin D. It is the only nutrient that is acquired through exposure to the sun, hence its nickname the "sunshine vitamin." Due to the massive and ongoing changes in lifestyle that industrialization has brought about, it could be that many people are deficient. Few people get enough sun exposure to generate adequate amounts of the vitamin throughout the year. Having good vitamin D levels is crucial for the health of the bones.[14] There is also an association with higher levels of circulating vitamin D in the blood and lowered risk of death due to cardiovascular disease, cancer, and other causes.[15]

There are two forms of the vitamin: D3 which is found mainly in animal products (good sources are fatty fish and egg yolks), and D2 which is found in some plants (good sources are mushrooms and yeast). Research suggests that vitamin D3 is better at increasing the level of calcifediol, the main circulating form of vitamin D, in the blood stream, and some studies have shown that due to diet, vegans might have lower levels and therefore decreased bone mineral density.[16]

Bone health isn't the only thing that vitamin D supports. The immune system, in particular, depends on vitamin D to function properly. After years of being deficient in vitamin D, many people develop inflammatory or autoimmune diseases. There is also some evidence that vitamin D increases upper and lower limb strength in healthy individuals.[17]

Vitamin D Recommended Dietary Allowance (RDA)[18]

Age	DRI (IU)
0–12 months	400 (10mcg)
1–70	600 (15 mcg)
70 and over	800 (20 mcg)
Pregnancy and breastfeeding	600 (15 mcg)

UPPING YOUR VITAMIN D INTAKE ON A PLANT-BASED DIET

There are a number of ways you can increase your vitamin D intake:

1. Make use of fortified products. There are a variety of foods fortified with vitamin D, such as dairy-free milk and yoghurt, cereals, and orange juice. Mushrooms are the best whole food plant-based source, but bear in mind, a cup of mushrooms will only be 1% of your DRI.

2. Make sure you get some sunshine twice a week. To boost vitamin D levels, expose the face, arms, legs, or back to the sun for five to thirty

minutes twice a week between 10 am and after 3 pm, without sunscreen. This is difficult if it's the winter and you're really far north or south.

3. Supplement your vitamin D intake. Vegans might need to supplement vitamin D if sun exposure and diet do not meet recommended levels. Always consult your physician before taking any supplements. Also bear in mind that there is an important distinction to be made between vitamin D3 (cholecalciferol) and vitamin D2 (ergocalciferol): vitamin D3 is usually derived from animals (lanolin), but vitamin D2 is made from yeast hence is acceptable for plant-based eaters.

CHOLINE

Choline is an essential nutrient. It is required for cognitive functions, cellular communication, and metabolism. An inadequate intake of choline may lead to high cholesterol levels and serious problems with the liver, heart, and brain.[19] Unfortunately the best sources of choline are meat and dairy. Eggs have a particularly high choline content. The nutrient is present in most plants, but usually in much smaller amounts.

Choline Adequate Intake (AI)

Age	Male	Female	Pregnancy	Breastfeeding
0 to 6 months	125 mg/day	125 mg/day		
7–12 months	150 mg/day	150 mg/day		
1–3 years	200 mg/day	200 mg/day		
4–8 years	250 mg/day	250 mg/day		
9–13 years	375 mg/day	375 mg/day		
14–18 years	550 mg/day	400 mg/day	450 mg/day	550 mg/day
19+ years	550 mg/day	425 mg/day	450 mg/day	550 mg/day

If you are eating a varied diet, even if it is strictly vegan, it is likely that you will get an adequate amount of choline. However, if you are heavily reliant on processed foods and eat a limited range of vegetables and no legumes, you may very well have a problem. This is a statement that applies to the important nutrients in any diet though!

Plant-Based Sources of Choline

Food	Serving	Choline (mg)
Almonds, dry roasted	1 oz	7
Apples, raw, with skin	1 large	8
Medjool dates	1	10
Flaxseed, ground	2 tbsp	11
Potatoes, boiled, in skin	½ cup	11
Bananas, raw	1 medium	12
Bread, whole wheat	1 slice	15
Peanuts	1 oz	15
Sunflower seeds	1 oz	15
Oranges, raw	1 large	16
Oats	1 cup	17
Brown rice, cooked	1 cup	18
Peanut butter, smooth	2 tbsp	20
Quinoa, uncooked	¼ cup	30
Soy milk, unfortified	1 cup	57
Broccoli, cooked	1 cup	63
Brussels sprouts, cooked	1 cup	63
Lentils, cooked	1 cup	65
Chickpeas, cooked	1 cup	70

A final note: one study of more than 47,000 men found that increased choline intake was associated with an increased risk of lethal prostate cancer, so although it is an essential nutrient, too much over a prolonged period time might not be good for your health. This could be due to the fact that foods highest in choline come from animal sources, and therefore contain the associated saturated fat and animal protein. Before you consider any kind of supplementation, it is important to speak to your health care provider.

IRON

About 4 grams of your bodyweight is iron. It may not seem like much – the same weight as about 4 paperclips – but that iron is critically important to your health. Proteins in red blood cells and muscles use iron to transport oxygen from the lungs to every part of the body. The mineral is also needed to produce thyroid hormones and low levels can cause fatigue and weakness. Deficiency can lead to anemia, a condition where your body does not produce enough red blood cells. This can be particularly problematic in children and can lead to behavioral problems and brain damage.[20]

Most people know that plants contain iron: the cartoon Popeye established the myth that spinach contains enough to give you big bulging muscles. However, if you are on a plant-based diet, you can face some unique difficulties in consuming enough. Research has shown that vegetarians and vegans have lower iron levels in their blood, and a higher proportion had iron-deficiency anemia, when compared to non-vegetarians.[21]

There are a couple of reasons why. Firstly, there are two types of iron found in food: heme iron, which is only found in meat, and non-heme, which is found in plants. Heme iron is easier to absorb than non-heme which must first be transformed into a soluble form before it can be used by the body. Secondly, vegans suffer from a decreased ability to absorb iron due to phytate and polyphenols, which are found in plant-based food. Phytate (also known as phytic acid), which is found in grains, legumes, nuts, beans, and seeds – basically most of the things that you eat as a vegan – inhibit the absorption of non-heme iron, as do the tannins in red wine, tea, and coffee.[22] These compounds bind to the iron and form insoluble compounds, preventing the iron being absorbed in the gut. Overall, this means that even though spinach, at 2.6mg per 100g, contains more iron than a sirloin steak, at 2.5mg per 100g, you absorb far less of the iron from the spinach – 1.7% compared to 20%. That translates to just 0.044 milligrams of iron from the spinach compared to 0.5 milligrams from the beef.[23] A pre-menopausal woman would have to eat almost 41kg of spinach a day to get the RDA of spinach in her a diet.

Recommended Dietary Allowances (RDA) for Iron

Age	Male (mg)	Female (mg)	Pregnancy	Breastfeeding
0–6 months	0.27 mg	0.27 mg		
7–12 months	11 mg	11 mg		
1–3 years	7 mg	7 mg		
4–8 years	10 mg	10 mg		
9–13 years	8 mg	8 mg		
14 - 18 years	11 mg	15 mg	27 mg	10 mg
19 - 50 years	8 mg	18 mg	27 mg	9 mg
51+	8 mg	8 mg		

If you are unfortunate to suffer from a gut disorder such as inflammatory bowel disease, celiac disease, Crohn's disease or even irritable bowel syndrome, this can also inhibit the absorption of iron. There is some evidence that calcium and zinc prevent iron from being absorbed in the gut effectively, so make sure you don't take a dietary supplement which contains them when you are eating iron-rich foods.

Due to the difficulty in absorbing iron on a plant-based diet, the Institute of Medicine in the USA recommends a higher RDA for iron than this – up to 1.8 times higher than for those who eat meat.[24]

Even without anemia, research shows that athletic performance is improved in those who are iron-deficient and receive supplementation.[25] In fact, requirements for athletes may be higher, especially if they participate in regular intense endurance exercise, up to 30-70% higher.[26] The upper limit for iron consumption in adults is 45 mg.

Plant-Based Sources of Iron

Food	Serving size	Amount (mg)
Tempeh, cooked	1 cup	4.5
Soybeans, cooked	1 cup	4.5
Kidney beans, cooked	1 cup	5.2
Spinach, cooked	1 cup	6.4
Lentils, cooked	1 cup	6.6
Tofu	½ cup	6.6

BOOSTING YOUR IRON INTAKE

Iron deficiency, whether it is with anemia or not, can have an impact on performance by impairing muscle function and limiting the amount of work you can do. If you suspect you may be iron deficient, seek medical advice.

There are some simple ways to increase the absorption of the iron that you get from your diet:

- Add foods containing vitamin C to your meals
- Avoid drinking tea, coffee, red wine and cocoa within an hour of eating a meal
- Don't take calcium supplements at mealtimes
- Follow some of the protocols below when preparing your food (see Countering the antinutrients)

Some medical professionals will recommend eating meat if you are vegan or vegetarian and have an iron deficiency. However, supplemental iron and vitamin C will be equally as effective to bring levels back up, so make sure you talk through all your choices.

CALCIUM

Calcium has a close relationship with vitamin D. It is also necessary for the development and maintenance of a healthy bone matrix. Calcium is the most abundant mineral in the body, largely stored in the bones and teeth, contributing to their strength and stability, accounting for about 1-2% of your total bodyweight. It also contributes to hormone secretion, nerve signaling, and maintaining proper heart rhythm as well as muscle contraction and blood clotting. Calcium stored in our bones supplies the balance in our blood and tissues if we do not get enough through our diet. Bones are constantly being remodeled, minerals removed or laid down, depending on the calcium needs of the body and the stress placed on the skeleton by our daily activities. It must be regularly replenished to prevent long term bone damage and loss. Research shows that low intake of calcium for boys during adolescence results in a lower adult height because the bones don't grow as large.[27]

Without the right levels of vitamin D, calcium cannot be adequately absorbed from the foods you eat. Just as with iron, some antinutrients also inhibit the absorption of calcium from the diet. Phytates, again, are a big culprit here, as is oxalic acid. You find oxalic acid in spinach, rhubarb, sweet potatoes, and beet greens. That means that when you eat spinach, for instance, you won't be able to absorb the totality of its fairly high calcium content.

High sodium in your diet can also reduce your calcium levels. When sodium levels in the blood are too high, the body gets rid of it by excreting it through the kidneys into the urine. However, calcium also goes with it, and lower levels of calcium in the blood means that more is taken from the bone matrix to use for the myriad other processes the mineral is needed for in the body.

The reference table below uses the figures that the USA and Canada recommend. These are similar to the recommendations from the World Health Organization. Europe opts for slightly lower numbers, and the UK for considerably less – only 700mg for most adults. Some research suggests that below 700mg per day, there is an increased risk of bone fracture and osteoporosis.[28]

Recommended Dietary Allowances (RDAs) for Calcium

Age	Male	Female	Pregnancy	Breastfeeding
0–6 months	200 mg	200 mg		
7–12 months	260 mg	260 mg		
1–3 years	700 mg	700 mg		
4–8 years	1000 mg	1000 mg		
9–13 years	1300 mg	1300 mg		
14–18 years	1300 mg	1300 mg	1300 mg	1300 mg
19–50 years	1000 mg	1000 mg	1000 mg	1000 mg
51–70 years	1000 mg	1200 mg		
70+ years	1200 mg	1200 mg		

Dairy products and fish with bones that you eat, like sardines, contain the highest levels of calcium. On a vegan diet, without eating fortified foods, it is hard to reach the RDA without careful planning. Soya products will be the easiest way to up your intake. A meta-analysis from 2009 determined that vegetarian and vegan diets are associated with lower bone mineral density.[29]

Plant-Based Sources of Calcium

Food	Serving size	Amount (mg)
Soy milk	1 cup	60
Orange	1 large	74
Kale, cooked	1 cup	94
Seaweed, nori	1 cup	126
Baked beans	1 cup	154
Bok choy, cooked	1 cup	158
Chia seeds	1 oz	179
Black-eyed peas	½ cup	185
Almonds	½ cup	189
Blackstrap molasses	1 tbsp	192
Chickpeas, cooked	1 cup	239
Dried figs	1 cup	241
Spinach, cooked	1 cup	243
Collard greens, cooked	1 cup	268
Soya beans, cooked	1 cup	515
Firm tofu	½ cup	861

CALCIUM SUPPLEMENTS

If your plant-based diet contains sufficient calcium from sources that are highly absorbable, you do not need to take calcium supplements. Those who struggle to meet the daily calcium requirements when following a plant-based diet may benefit from taking a vegan calcium supplement. Calcium supplements have drawn some concern over their safety. The research suggests that high doses may cause side effects, so supplements shouldn't be the only source of calcium.[30] Calcium supplements in small doses should not cause harm and could serve as a good boost to vegan diets that lack calcium, although you should consult your physician before beginning to take any supplements. You should always remember that most nutrients (including calcium) have an upper intake level. For adults it's 2,500 mg of calcium from dietary sources and supplements combined.

A short note on bone health

Despite what the ads told us in the 1980s, you don't need to drink milk to have strong bones. The simplest and best advice for maintaining healthy bones, especially as you age, is to do to resistance training. If the tissues of your bones are exposed to mechanical loads which are greater than they receive through day-to-day living, this will usually result in bone mass accretion. It doesn't have to be resistance training – jumping or hopping will work for your lower limbs – but using weights is usually the most straight forward method.

ZINC

Zinc is an essential mineral. Its primary function is to act as an enzyme cofactor, and it is involved in at least fifty biochemical reactions in the human body. One of the key signs of zinc deficiency is an impaired immune system, and also loss of appetite. If it is particularly severe, there can be weight loss, loss of hair, and delayed healing of wounds. A lack of zinc can impair cell growth. Therefore, it is essential to have enough zinc during pregnancy and for growing children; also, as zinc is needed for testosterone and sperm production, males require more in their diet than females.

Recommended Dietary Allowances (RDAs) for Zinc

Age	Male (mg)	Female (mg)	Pregnancy	Breastfeeding
0–6 months	2 mg	2 mg		
7–12 months	3 mg	3 mg		
1–3 years	3 mg	3 mg		
4–8 years	5 mg	5 mg		
9–13 years	8 mg	8 mg		
14 - 18 years	11 mg	9 mg	12 mg	13 mg
19+	11 mg	8 mg	11 mg	12 mg
51+	8 mg	8 mg		

The research is mixed as to whether vegetarians and vegans are getting enough zinc in their diet, although large studies and reviews point towards lower intakes, which is why we have included it in this chapter. Both a 2013 meta-analysis of 34 studies[31] and a 30,000-participant study into cancer which included zinc intakes[32] suggested that dietary consumption and therefore blood serum levels were significantly lower in vegetarian diets.

In a diet that uses animal products, meat and shellfish are where you'd get most of your zinc. In a plant-based diet, it comes from grains, legumes, seeds, and nuts. As with iron and calcium, phytates in these foods can limit the absorbability of the mineral, and plant-based eaters are recommended to try to get 1.5 times the RDA of the mineral in their diet.[33]

Plant-Based Sources of Zinc

Food	Serving size	Amount (mg)
Cashews, raw	33 g	1.91
Chia seeds	43 g	1.98
Tofu, firm	266 g	2.21
Sesame seeds	38 g	2.56
Chickpeas, boiled	170 g	2.65
Lentils, boiled	209 g	2.66
Pumpkin seeds	35 g	2.73
Oatmeal, dry	100 g	2.98
Hemp seeds, hulled	40 g	3.69
Buckwheat, dry	180 g	4.31

A short note on cadmium (and zinc supplementation)

Some studies have linked vegan diets to higher levels of cadmium. Cadmium is a heavy metal that is commonly found in the soil and is toxic to human health. It can cause a lot of problems, from kidney disease to diabetes and cancer. One theory is that because cadmium is stored in the bran of grains, increased consumption of whole grains in a vegan diet might lead to higher levels in the blood.[34]

The best solution isn't to stop eating whole grains, or even to check the cadmium levels of the soil in which your produce is grown (although if you're growing your own, that is something you can do). The best solution could be to take a zinc supplement. Deficiencies in both iron and zinc increase the absorption of cadmium, and in particular, zinc boosts the level of a mineral-binding protein that prevents cadmium from being damaging to the body. In fact, zinc supplementation has been linked to a systemic anti-inflammatory effect and the reduced risk of breast cancer.[35]

COUNTERING THE ANTINUTRIENTS

It can seem a bit unfair to refer to these compounds as "antinutrients" when they can also have a positive effect on human health. For instance, tannins have been found to have anticarcinogenic properties, and to be antimicrobial as well. They are referred to as antinutrients because they reduce the body's ability to absorb some key nutrients, like iron, calcium and zinc as we've discussed above, and they're found in particularly high concentrations in seeds, nuts, legumes and grains.

It is possible to lightly process foods to reduce the effects of the antinutrients, and these are techniques that have been used since the dawn of modern agriculture. They are:

- Soaking - usually overnight.
- Sprouting - where you start the germination process in the seed, grain or legume.
- Fermentation - where you try and use microorganisms to digest some of the carbohydrates in the food – like in sourdough bread.
- Boiling

Using a combination of the techniques is usually most effective. For instance, you'll often start with soaking before doing anything else. Here's a brief breakdown of the main antinutrients and how to mitigate their effects:

Phytate (phytic acid): particularly high in bran (found in whole grain rice and wheat) and almonds, phytate is found in all seeds, nuts, grains and beans. Soaking, sprouting and fermentation are the best ways to break it down.

Lectins: found in all plants, especially nightshade vegetables (tomatoes, peppers, eggplant), legumes (including peanut products). Soaking, boiling and fermentation break down lectins, as does heating of any sort.

Protease inhibitors: found in a wide variety of plants, including most grains and legumes, but also some fruit and vegetables. They can affect the digestion of protein and can be broken down by soaking, sprouting and boiling.

Tannins: found in most legumes – red-colored beans have the highest content. They can be reduced by soaking and boiling.

Oxalate (oxalic acid): found in plants (especially leafy greens, some vegetables, fruits, nuts and seeds). The oxalic acid binds to calcium to form calcium oxalate which isn't absorbed when you eat the foods which contain it. It can be reduced by soaking and boiling.

IODINE

The body cannot produce iodine itself, making it an essential mineral. The main reason that iodine is so important is that it plays a role in the formation of thyroid hormones. Thyroid hormones are vital for proper brain and bone development. They control metabolism in the body and deficiencies can cause hypothyroidism and other health problems. The effects of this over time may result in an enlarged thyroid, also known as a goiter. Due to its critical role in growth and development, iodine plays a particularly important role in pregnant mothers and children.

In developing countries, one of the most common nutritional deficiencies is for iodine. In many western countries, the introduction of iodized salt has meant that deficiency is less widespread. In an omnivorous diet, iodine's major sources are dairy products and seafood.

In addition to the fact that strict vegans do not consume either dairy products or seafood, people are generally encouraged to limit their sodium intake and therefore eat less salt. This might make it challenging to ensure enough iodine is absorbed on a vegan diet.

Recommended Dietary Allowances (RDA) for Iodine

Age	Male (mcg)	Female (mcg)	Pregnancy	Breastfeeding
0–6 months	110 mcg	110 mcg		
7–12 months	130 mcg	130 mcg		
1–3 years	90 mcg	90 mcg		
4–8 years	90 mcg	90 mcg		
9–13 years	120 mcg	120 mcg		
14 - 18 years	150 mcg	150 mcg	220 mcg	290 mcg
19+	150 mcg	150 mcg	220 mcg	290 mcg

Most research points to vegans having a low intake of iodine in their diet.[36] However, it is hard to determine as the methods for measuring intake (usually from iodine content in the urine) are subject to problems within the research methodology. When you look at thyroid health, then vegans tend to have normal levels of thyroid stimulating hormone, thyroxine, hyperthyroidism and hypothyroidism.[37] In other words, the research is conflicting, but the fact that vegans have normal thyroid function suggests that iodine deficiency is not a problem.

Levels of iodine in the soil will determine how much will end up in the plants that grow from that soil. Levels are much higher nearer the coast than they are inland, so where you get your vegetables from will make a difference to your iodine intake.

Plant-Based Sources of Iodine

Food	Serving size	Amount (mcg)
Green beans	½ cup	3
Bananas	1 medium	3
Strawberries	1 cup	13
Prunes	5 whole	13
Corn	½ cup	14
Navy beans	½ cup	32
Potato	1 medium	60
Cranberries	4 oz	400
Alaria	¼ oz	1162
Dulse	¼ oz	1169
Kelp	¼ oz	3170

Bear in mind that there are also some foods that interfere with the absorption of iodine from the diet. These are foods which contain goitrogens, such as soy, flax seed and cruciferous vegetables, like broccoli, cauliflower and cabbage. If your iodine intake is adequate, consumption of these foods is unlikely to cause you problems. However, if it is consistently lower than the RDA, it might be a good idea to take a supplement, especially if your diet relies heavily on goitrogen-containing foods.

THE LONG TERM

Fine tuning your micronutrients takes time. Don't get overwhelmed by all the numbers and tables. If you're really concerned about clinical deficiencies, then you should speak to your healthcare provider and get blood tests if appropriate. Most people won't have a problem with a deficiency, but their intake of one or more micronutrients might not be at the best level to ensure your body can perform at its best.

If you're new to a plant-based diet, then sub-optimal levels of micronutrients will take longer to show up. If you've been vegan for a long time and haven't paid much attention to the quantity of iron or calcium that you eat, or any of the items covered in this chapter, then it is a good idea to make an assessment of your current diet and work out what might need boosting. You might find a small change will really help.

Nutrition is for the long term – getting it right won't be a quick fix. This has benefits and disadvantages. The hard part is that it takes time and effort, but because it takes time, day-to-day decisions can be easily adjusted. Eating food which doesn't contain the optimal levels of specific micronutrients on one day won't derail the whole plan – even a few days won't change long-term outcomes much. Once you've been following a plan consistently for several weeks, then you can begin to see how to make the right kind of adjustments.

CHAPTER 9

PUSHING UP PERFORMANCE

I've found that taking shortcuts will get you to the place you don't want to be much quicker than they get u to the place u want to be

Lennox Lewis

Will cutting out meat make a difference? That's the big question that I often get asked by people who are thinking of adopting more of a plant-based lifestyle. Will it affect their ability to train as hard as they would like to? In other words, they're not too worried about their baseline health, but rather whether they might be missing something in meat or dairy that will give them a performance edge.

As a vegan or vegetarian, there are several nutrients that you do not ordinarily get in your diet, which research shows might have some benefit. As always, with nutrition, the information is double edged – the possible benefit you might get must be weighed up against the potential downsides, not least that you might not get any benefit at all.

CREATINE

Creatine is important for improving endurance, strength, and mental sharpness. It plays a role in the body's energy systems (see Chapter 5), where it is stored in the muscles in a phosphorylated form as a short-term source of energy.

In a diet that relies on animal products, that's where you'd get creatine from – storage in the muscle that the animal was intending to use for its own energy. Therefore, for plant-based eaters, creatine can come from 2 sources:

- Endogenously - The liver produces approximately 1g of creatine a day from amino acids arginine, glycine, and methionine.

- Creatine supplementation – You can take creatine monohydrate as a supplement.

Vegetarians can obtain some creatine from eggs and dairy, but not in large quantities. Vegans and vegetarians are found to have lower creatine stores, which makes sense because of their relatively low dietary intakes.[1]

In general, a low dietary intake will not cause deficiency. It's only if your endogenous creatine production or storage is reduced by a medical condition that you may experience a clinical deficiency.

CREATINE SUPPLEMENTATION

Creatine is one of the most popular supplements for muscle building in the world for vegans and omnivores alike. I recommend it to clients if they are following a challenging training regime regardless of their dietary preferences. However, it is of particular benefit to plant-based eaters. One study saw that vegetarians had enhanced physical performance and developed more lean muscle tissue when compared to nonvegetarians when they both took creatine supplements.[2] It has also been shown that vegetarians who take creatine supplements have enhanced memory, cognitive ability, and overall intelligence.[3]

So, for an average person, adding creatine supplements is not so much about preventing deficiencies but more about improving athletic and potentially cognitive performance. It appears to be safe to take for those who do not have a history of kidney disease. The International Society of Sports Nutrition recommends 5g of creatine monohydrate taken 4 times a day for 5-7 days as the most effective way of increasing stores of creatine in the muscles.[4] No side effects have been found from taking 20g/day for longer – up to 5 weeks – but longer than that has not been studied. Anecdotally, I haven't heard of anyone having problems with supplementing creatine for more than 5 weeks.

CARNITINE

The molecule carnitine contributes to the metabolism of fatty acids, allowing cells to use fat for energy.[5] Carnitine in the form L-carnitine is found mainly in meat, and vegetarians are usually found to have lower levels of it in the blood. Some studies have also shown that vegetarians also have lower levels of muscle carnitine, as well as reduced capabilities for transporting carnitine to muscle cells.[6]

Carnitine deficiency in skeletal muscles results in a severe muscle dysfunction, which is the rationale behind why this nutrient has sometimes been used as a supplement to improve athletic performance. However, studies on the effects of carnitine supplementation on exercise and performance have been inconclusive. There is some evidence that supplementing it in rats has positive effects on their metabolism, but this has not translated to human athletic performance.[7]

Although vegans and vegetarians consume little dietary carnitine, they can still rely on their own natural production to avoid deficiency, as long as they are consuming the required precursors. Be sure to get enough protein, iron, vitamin C, and B vitamins in your diet so that your body can produce the necessary amount of carnitine.

TAURINE

One of the ingredients in the energy drink Red Bull, Taurine is often referred to as an amino acid, although it is actually an amino sulfonic acid. It is not essential, but conditionally essential. Normally the body can produce enough for its physiological requirements, however, under certain conditions, like extreme illness or other physiologically stressful situations, the body might not be able to produce an adequate supply. It is found in all animal tissues, in greatest concentrations in the brain, heart, eyes and muscles. It is responsible for a wide variety of biochemical actions, including muscle function, antioxidation, and the production of bile salts. It also plays a key role in regulating the stress response.

Non-vegetarians eat between 40 and 70 milligrams of taurine a day, and without meat in their diet, vegans usually have measurably lower levels of taurine in the blood. Even though taurine isn't found in plant-based food, the body is capable of producing it on its own. Moreover, when taurine levels are low, the body is able to conserve it as a lower amount is excreted in the urine. So, it is highly unlikely that you'll become deficient.

There is mixed evidence that taurine will improve athletic performance by reducing fatigue, muscle damage, and recovery times, whilst increasing strength and power.[8] More research is needed for conclusive evidence though, because the results tend to be small and inconsistent.

CARNOSINE

As an antioxidant contained in the muscles and the brain, carnosine is known to enhance longevity.[9] It is mainly found in meat and, to a lesser extent, dairy products which is why vegetarians often have lower levels of carnosine in their muscles. The amino acids histidine and beta-alanine are required for your body to produce carnosine, so it is not an essential nutrient, and you are unlikely to become deficient in it. However, studies have shown that carnosine levels can affect performance – high levels of carnosine in the muscles are linked to decreased muscle fatigue.[10] It acts as a buffer for acid and can help to counteract the effects of the elevated levels of lactic acid produced in the muscles during intense training.

As there are no plants that can provide carnosine, vegans can add a beta-alanine supplement to their diet, to make sure that enough is produced in the body.

COLLAGEN

Collagen is one of the proteins that makes up a lot of the connective tissues in animals. It is made up of non-essential amino acids, so the body is able to produce it. However, there is some evidence that supplementing collagen can be beneficial for those suffering from knee osteoarthritis, especially if they have a low meat intake. This is why we've included it in this section. Joint damage can severely limit performance, and taking collagen seems to reduce subjective assessment of joint pain in the knees. How far this reduction goes needs further study. The research is quite mixed – a couple of studies found that supplementing collagen helped reduced joint pain in college athletes after exercising, but another found that the only reduction in knee pain was from those diagnosed with osteoarthritis of the knee.[11] There are vegan sources of collagen available, and it may be something worth considering, depending on the state of your joints.

THE SUPPLEMENT SOLUTION

You can get a bit carried away with supplements. It's easy to think that they're the secret solution to why you're not as fast or as strong or as lean as you want to be. Usually it's all marketing, hype and some sketchy science. Setting up a proper nutrition plan and a good training program will always be the most important actions you can take to improve your performance.

At one point or another, I've tried them all – except for collagen, and I'm sure I'll try that if my knees start hurting! Creatine has been the only one that I've gone back to again and again. If you're supplementing vitamin B12 (which I highly recommend – see Chapter 8 if you haven't already) it's easy to add another supplement to your routine to see how you fare on it. You might find extra carnitine or taurine gives you the boost that you need, or you might find after a few weeks it feels like it's doing nothing at all. Don't try them all at once, be systematic during the testing phase. You have to find out what works for you. Research often gives mixed results because the sample size that's used is too small. And remember: everyone's different. You might find one of these supplements is exactly what you've been missing.

One of the big reasons why everyone's different – at least from the effect that nutrition has on their biochemistry – is because of the gut. That's what we're going to cover in the next chapter, the amazing interactions that the microbiome creates.

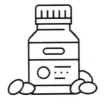

CHAPTER 10

IT'S ALWAYS ABOUT THE GUT

All diseases begin in the gut.

Hippocrates

It's impossible to write a book about nutrition and not mention the gut. You can exactly calculate the different kinds of nutrients that your food contains, you can plan your diet very precisely based on RDAs and DVs, but it is very unlikely that you'll know what actually happens to those nutrients after you've eaten them. How much are absorbed from your food is down to the composition of your gut microbiome, and unless you sample it and sequence its genome, which few people do, you have no way of knowing what it contains. By now, most people have some inkling of the impact of the gut on human health. It's been used to sell yogurt so consistently, that many people are at least aware of the idea of "good bacteria." Now we're beginning to understand the far-reaching effects of all the bacteria, good or otherwise.

It seems amazing that for so many years, nutrition science concentrated on the nutrients contained within the food, and how these nutrients were used by the cells of the body, but not on the point of transfer between the food and the body – the gut. Now we're catching up, as more research is unearthing new discoveries, helping us understand the remarkable connections it makes.

WHAT IS THE GUT MICROBIOME?

There are trillions of bacteria and their genetic material living in your intestinal tract, collectively known as your gut microbiome. This group of microorganisms, weighing about 2.5kg and mainly composed of bacteria, but also containing viruses, fungi and protozoa, plays a critical role in your health and well-being. You contain about 10 times more cells from other organisms compared to human cells, hosting approximately 1,000 different species of bacteria in your gut. They play a vital role in digesting the food you consume and facilitate the absorption of nutrients. But they also play a role in their synthesis: vitamins, and short-chain fatty acids are produced by these bacteria. Furthermore, they play a vital role in other functions that extend beyond the digestive system, such as metabolism, weight control, immune function, mental and physical health.

At an early age, bacteria begin to populate your gut - there is even some suggestion that this process begins while the fetus is still developing.[1] The types of bacteria in your gut depend on various factors such as your genetics and the health of your parents, whether you were born from a vaginal or cesarean delivery, whether you were breastfed or bottle-fed, and of course, what you eat on a regular basis. The populations of bacteria that live in your gut continue to be shaped by a variety of factors as you grow. It is difficult to change some of these factors, such as genetics, stressful events, or illnesses, but it is possible to change certain behaviors, such as our lifestyles and diet.

WHAT DOES A HEALTHY GUT LOOK LIKE?

The inside surface of the intestines constitutes a much greater surface area than the surface of your skin. The surface area of the small intestine which is effectively in contact with the external environment – the food that you put into your body – is about 250m2, compared to the 2m2 of the skin. The intestines must do two things simultaneously: allow beneficial nutrients into the blood stream while preventing toxins and microorganisms from entering. A healthy gut possesses a complex barrier capable of performing these two opposing functions.

In fact, it's such a smart system that it allows a low level of bacterial translocation from the intestine through to the lymph nodes to act as a kind of training ground for the immune system, in case of a big invasion of pathogens. The immune system is one layer of the gut barrier

– there is also the mechanical barrier made up of cells which line the intestinal tract, as well as the barrier that the gut flora provides.

Based on existing evidence, having a wide range of diverse types of bacteria living in your gut is considered beneficial. Reduction in diversity is associated with increases in human disease. With a wider range of bacteria in your gut, it may be more equipped to combat and resist pathogens due to this diversity – in simple terms, the good bacteria compete for space and nutrients with pathogenic ones, and the more populations of good bacteria that you have, the stronger that defense will be. Moreover, if one strain of bacteria cannot perform its task, another of a similar type can step in to complete it.[2]

The food you eat plays a big part in the composition of the microbiome, but other factors also seem to be incredibly important: exercise, sleep and stress levels.

SYMPTOMS OF AN UNHEALTHY GUT

You know intuitively what a healthy gut feels like because its smooth operation is so central to your overall feeling of wellbeing. However, you don't have access to the ecosystem within your gut, you can only experience the downstream effects of any problems it might have. Long-term effects of an unhealthy gut can be wide-ranging and have been linked to some serious conditions like autoimmune and endocrine disorders, cardiovascular disease and cancer. Here are some symptoms of an unhealthy gut that you might notice:

Discomfort in the abdomen: This is the obvious one. Any kind of stomach upset, like diarrhea or constipation, bloating or gas is usually a sign of an imbalance of some sort, although usually short-lived. Start to recognize which foods cause which kind of reaction in your gut and notice if a pattern emerges.

Sleep problems: If you're having very broken sleep, it could be a sign of an imbalance in your gut. Research is not clear on the exact causes, but there is strong connection between sleep quality and the microbiome. One suggested mechanism is that the bacteria in the gut create a kind of internal clock due to the chemicals they produce through metabolism.[3]

Mood fluctuations: You respond to stressful situations better when your gut microbiome is functioning well. Gut health plays a significant role in mood changes, partly due to the connection between the brain and the gut. Known as the gut-brain axis, several communication routes enable the gut and brain to communicate with each other. It's a two-way street. When you feel butterflies in the stomach because an upcoming event has been stressing you out, it could be that the brain is sending signals that are felt in the gut. But it also works in reverse: changes and imbalances in the microbiome may result in anxiety and mood disorders.

A whole host of neurochemicals are produced by gut bacteria that regulate specific physiological processes, including mood, memory, and learning. A significant portion of the body's serotonin is produced by gut bacteria, which plays a part both in mood regulation and digestive function.[4]

Skin problems: The skin has a microbiome of its own, and this is affected by the gut. The gut-skin axis, which is mediated by the immune system, plays a significant role in skin health. Changes to the skin, like the onset of dermatitis, psoriasis, acne or dandruff, might be a sign of an imbalance in the gut.[5]

Insufficient immunity: The gut contains about 70% of the immune system. Poor gut health can lead to poor immune function and illness.[6] As we discussed above, the gut barrier plays a crucial role in immune response and researchers have also found that changes in gut microbes can result in more serious immune dysregulation, which might lead to autoimmune disorders.[7]

A PLANT-BASED DIET AND GUT HEALTH

A plant-based diet appears to be beneficial for gut health because it increases the diversity of the microbiome. The key to understanding the mechanisms behind this is that the bacteria which thrive are the ones that are fed. If you eat a diverse plant-based diet that contains a lot of fermentable fiber, it will encourage diverse bacterial growth. If you feed them, bacterial populations will increase, if they aren't fed regularly, they will shrink.

For instance, Lactobacillus, which breaks down sugars from dairy products, is common in the guts of people who easily digest milk. Lactobacillus will die off if you do not consume dairy products for a long period of time and it will mean that your gut will be unable to handle dairy if you abruptly start eating it again.[8]

The research is not always completely clear, and it is ongoing. In a pivotal study, researchers studied the gut bacteria of European and rural African children. In comparison to African children, European children ate a largely western diet that included a lot of processed foods, while African children consumed a fiber-rich rural diet that mostly consisted of plant-based foods. Results showed a stark difference between the gut bacteria of the two groups. In general, the African children had more types of bacteria, many of which were anti-inflammatory, lowering the long-term risk of disease associated with harmful inflammation. In the European group, there were far fewer types of healthy bacteria.[9] This was a small study with only 14 African children and 15 Italian children, but a larger study – with 101 adults (so still quite small) – showed that vegetarians also have a greater richness of microbiota than omnivores. However, although there was more diversity, the study suggested that the actual composition of the different microbiomes and whether they were full of beneficial bacteria or not might be more influenced by the quality of the diet. Rather than resting on whether the diet was plant-based or not, how much processed food, fat and sugar it contained determined gut health, rather than whether it is plant-based or not.[10] That means vegan junk food will probably be as bad for your gut as non-vegan junk food. The bottom line is that the WFPB diet wins in terms of gut health.

PLANT-BASED DIETS AND GUT ISSUES

However, while a plant-based diet rich in fiber may have its benefits, it can be problematic when you are first starting out. Here are some of the reasons why:

Increased fiber intake

If you make a big change from a typical Western diet (or the 'SAD' - Standard American Diet) with very little fiber to a vegetarian or vegan diet, this will lead to a significant increase in fiber intake. This has a lot of positive impact as we discussed in Chapter 5: reduced risk of type 2 diabetes, cardiovascular disease and colon cancer to name the most life changing.

Nevertheless, you may not become accustomed to it immediately – and in some cases high-fiber diets can promote gastric distress. On a basic level that everyone can identify with, fiber fermenting produces gas which isn't bad for you, but can cause discomfort, and will likely affect performance levels in the short term. If you're transitioning from an omnivorous diet to a plant-based diet, and your carbohydrate requirements are particularly high, you can include some lower fiber foods, like white rice and pasta, and remove the skins from tubers and root vegetables as this might help. I know quite a few people who have fallen at this hurdle – they introduced too much fiber too quickly and decided a plant-based diet was not for them. I always caution my clients to monitor how much extra fiber they are eating and to only increase it slowly if they feel it's causing them discomfort.

Make sure you drink enough water. Herbal teas like ginger, fennel and mint can also have a soothing effect on the digestive tract whilst providing hydration.

An increase intake of FODMAPs

If you suffer from irritable bowel syndrome (IBS), it is likely that you know what FODMAPs are. The acronym stands for Fermentable Oligosaccharides, Disaccharides, Monosaccharides, and Polyols, which are types of carbohydrate that can be poorly absorbed by the intestines. They travel to the large intestine where they are fermented by gut bacteria, causing gastrointestinal symptoms. If you suffer from IBS, it's likely that you have sensitivity to some FODMAPs.

The difficulty on a vegan diet, is that not only are a lot of plant-based protein sources, like grains and legumes, naturally high in FODMAPs, but also a lot of the other foods you might eat are too, like fruit. You can minimize the issue by making sure to include plenty of low-FODMAP foods in your diet, such as leafy greens, tomatoes, bananas, and potatoes. However, if you have sensitivity to some FODMAP-containing foods, you will need to carefully plan your diet to make sure you avoid them while still getting the right balance of macronutrients.

Gluten sensitivity

Gluten sensitivity is a condition in which you might experience gastrointestinal symptoms after consuming gluten, a protein found in wheat, barley and rye. These symptoms include bloating, abdominal pain, diarrhea, and constipation. It is not the same as Celiac disease, where your immune system attacks the lining of your gut when you eat gluten, which is a much more serious condition. Celiac disease affects about 1% of the US population, compared to up to 6% for gluten sensitivity.[11] While the exact cause of gluten sensitivity is unknown, it is believed to be related to the body's inability to properly break down gluten proteins. Since plant-based diets are often rich in gluten-containing grains, if you have gluten sensitivity or intolerance, you will have to plan your diet carefully.

WHAT CAN YOU DO TO MAXIMIZE GUT HEALTH?

Some dietary changes can be made to ensure that you are providing your gut bacteria with everything they need. Here are a few suggestions:

Eat whole grains

Unless you have a gluten sensitivity, this isn't exactly surprising advice – we've covered the health potential of whole grains before. In gut terms, beta-glucan and other nondigestible carbohydrates are found in whole grains; by not being absorbed in the small intestine, these carbohydrates can promote the growth of beneficial bacteria such as Bifidobacterium, Lactobacillus, and Bacteroidetes, in the large intestine.

Eat other prebiotic foods

Prebiotics are food ingredients that stimulate the growth of good bacteria in the gut. Generally, they are fibers or complex carbohydrates that the human body cannot digest and are broken down and used as fuel by specific species of bacteria in the gut.

However, getting more prebiotics in your diet is more than just saying eat more fiber! Some high-fiber food has higher quantities of prebiotic fiber than others. Particularly good sources are Jerusalem artichokes (sunchokes), garlic, onions, leeks, asparagus, bananas, apples, oats and barley. Try and vary your sources of this kind of gut food.

Eat probiotics

These are the foods which contain live healthy bacteria that transfer to your gut when you eat them. Anything fermented will be beneficial: sauerkraut, kimchi, pickled vegetables, kombucha, tempeh, water kefir and miso. It's a good idea to have a container of sauerkraut (or kimchi if you prefer) in your fridge so that you can have a forkful of it with your lunch or dinner. That way you will ensure a steady supply of probiotics in your diet, especially as cooked food like tempeh or miso usually loses all of its probiotics.

Eat a diverse diet

The "eat the rainbow" cliché has stuck around for a reason. Not only do different colored plants contain important phytochemicals and flavonoids, but if you try to eat as many different colored foods as you can, you'll end up eating lots of different things. The greater the diversity of foods in your diet, the greater the diversity of the gut microbiota, which has been strongly linked to good health. Try and regularly eat things that you don't normally eat – there are so many different types of food to try!

WRITE IT DOWN!

One of the simplest but most effective things you can do for your long-term nutrition is to keep a record. This can be as simple as just writing down what you've eaten during the day. If you're planning your meals carefully, you will probably already have it written down in advance. Try and keep some other notes with the food record: how well you slept, your mood, and how your gut feels. It doesn't have to be like keeping a journal unless you want it to be. Use numbers, emojis, or your own notation to keep it simple if you're short on time. That way you can track the effects of any changes in your diet, and you will start to notice how certain foods might be influencing your gut health.

You can also keep track of *when* you eat, because the timing of your food can have a big effect on long-term health and short-term performance. This is the subject of the next chapter.

CHAPTER 11

TIMING IS EVERYTHING

Think in the morning. Act in the noon. Eat in the evening. Sleep in the night.

William Blake

It turns out that this advice from William Blake – the part about eating at least – is back to front. Peak performance is all about timing. You can have a meticulously planned diet containing optimal amounts of both macro and micronutrients, but if it's not supplying you with the right amount of energy when you need it, or allowing you to recover in time, all that planning is for nothing. The bottom line is that you need your diet to ensure that you can perform, whether that's thinking, acting, or working out.

For some of my clients, paying attention to when they eat has been the biggest factor in making a sustainable change to their diet in the long term. For some, making just one simple change – not eating late at night – has completely changed their life. This chapter will look at three big questions in relation to timing: what should you eat *before*, *during* and *after* you train? This will shed light on how meal timing influences serious health outcomes, and how to make sure you can maintain your wellbeing throughout your entire life just by paying attention to when you eat.

SHOULD YOU EAT BEFORE EXERCISE?

This is a personal choice and depends a lot on both what outcomes you are looking for and what kind of exercise you're doing.

There is good evidence that if you're in a fasted state (you haven't eaten for 12-hours – for instance, if you've just woken up after a night's sleep), ingesting carbohydrates pre-workout will significantly improve your performance.[1] A pre-workout meal will replenish glycogen stores, so that muscles have an immediate source of energy.

However, there is also evidence that training in a fasted state provides beneficial metabolic adaptions that you wouldn't get if you ate some carbs just before the workout.[2] That means, if you're working out for weight management, to burn fat or to improve insulin sensitivity, then training in a fasted state may be beneficial.

WHEN SHOULD YOU EAT?

Ideally, you should consume a complete meal containing carbs, protein, and fat 2–3 hours before exercising to maximize your results. Remember that the closer you eat to your workout, the easier to digest the food needs to be. When you eat only 45-60 minutes prior to working out, aim for simple-to-digest foods rich in carbohydrates and protein. In this way, you will lower the possibility of gastrointestinal discomfort or stomach cramps while exercising.

Many studies have found that eating carbohydrates at least 60 minutes before exercise improved performance by 7-20%.[3] Another double-blind placebo-controlled study found that ingesting carbo-hydrates 30 minutes before exercise compared to 90 minutes provided a greater increase in exercise capacity.[4]

WHAT SHOULD YOU EAT?

It's hard to give specific advice about quantities or sources of pre-workout foods – you have to work out what works for you by experimentation. The challenge of determining how much to eat can be frustrating, and lead to some sub-optimal training sessions, but success depends on self-experimentation. Again, here the practice of keeping a record is very useful. During various levels of training intensity, you should try out different pre-workout meals and see what works best. If you're experimenting with nutrition protocols for a specific event, you should closely simulate conditions of the day of the event (time of day, environmental conditions, intensity) to achieve the best results.

Carbohydrates: These are the obvious choice: you need fuel. Glycogen is your muscles' most important source of energy during short-term and high-intensity exercise; your output and intensity decrease as glycogen stores are depleted.

Prolonged periods of exercise (over 60 minutes) done at moderate to high intensity (65–80% VO2max) will seriously deplete your internal stores. That means to maintain best performance you need a nutrition strategy that will maximize their replenishment. One method is carbohydrate loading – which can increase glycogen storage in muscles by up to 100%. This must happen over a period of several days during the week before an event, where for several days you eat 8-12g of carbohydrate per kg of bodyweight, cutting back on fats to maintain an energy balance.

Protein: Depending on what kind of training you are undertaking protein consumption may be a good idea too. Although most of the studies have been done with animal-based proteins, like whey, it seems likely that the effects will be similar with soy protein. There is plenty of evidence to suggest that eating a combination of protein and carbohydrates pre-exercise improves endurance. It also increases power output for resistance training. Protein on its own definitely stimulates muscle protein synthesis, but not more than if you ate it after a workout.[5]

Fats: There's no need to specifically consume high-fat foods before exercise. Your body has fat stores that it will start to use when you exercise for longer periods at a moderate to low intensity. No studies have been done specifically on pre-exercise fat consumption, mainly because it doesn't affect performance in the same way as carbohydrates.

EATING WHILE YOU WORK

Whether this is something you want to do will depend on both the type of exercise you're doing and your long-term goals.

Most research suggests that for prolonged bouts of aerobic exercise, ingesting carbohydrates during exercise will increase performance, and this performance increase is enhanced by higher frequency of consumption, for instance at 30-minute rather than 60-minute intervals. There are mixed findings over whether consuming carbs in the latter half of the exercise bout will be detrimental or not, and equally mixed results over whether ingesting carbohydrates during exercise with a duration of less than 90 minutes is beneficial at all.[6]

So, for short or high intensity exercise, eating during the event doesn't make any sense. You wouldn't try to swallow an energy drink in the 100m sprint. If performance isn't an issue – you're going for a long leisurely cycle ride – it isn't an issue either. Longer endurance exercise is where it makes the most sense – marathons, triathlons and distance hiking.

If you're looking to lose weight, you want to maximize your body's ability to metabolize fat stores. These will be used by the body to generate energy during aerobic exercise, so don't give yourself another fuel source if you want that to happen.

POST-WORKOUT NUTRITION

This has long been a hot topic of debate, and many people swear by a particular strategy. I've long been a big believer in making sure I have something straight after my main training session of the day – often a vegan post-workout shake that provides a mixture of protein and carbohydrates, or a well-balanced meal. However, as always, the research is mixed and it depends a lot on what sort of outcomes you're trying to achieve, and what sort of exercise you've just done.

WHEN AND WHAT SHOULD YOU EAT?

It is a compelling idea to think that there is a window of opportunity just after you've trained during which the body is in an ideal state to absorb nutrients. If you've done a hard workout, you certainly feel like you need refueling. In the gym, the timing you'll hear most often from trainers or muscle heads is that the window is 15-60 minutes after exercising.

Carbohydrates: Consuming carbohydrates within 30-60 minutes after exercise results in a higher rate of glycogen storage in the muscles than if you wait for 2 hours – it's 50% faster and more complete.[7] There is also some evidence that eating carbohydrates after prolonged endurance exercise creates a more favorable hormonal environment in the body with lower markers of inflammation.[8]

Bear in mind, that the timing of carbohydrate consumption is the most important if your main goal is to replenish glycogen stores as quickly as possible. For instance, if you're going to train again or are participating in an event that requires continuous activity, like a competition with rounds that take place throughout the course of a day.

If you're really serious about restoring levels of glycogen quickly after exhaustive exercise, then (≥ 1.2 g/kg/h) for four to six hours afterwards is the recommendation. That's a lot – for me it would amount to 2 and a half servings of whole wheat pasta per hour, which I've never done, and am not sure I want to.

If you're eating less than 1.2 g/kg/h of carbohydrates, then adding a bit of protein actually increases the rate of glycogen resynthesis. In fact, adding protein to your carbs after a workout increases insulin secretion which will promote the synthesis of glycogen, which is what you want.

For most people, eating your regular meals will restore glycogen levels as long as your daily carbohydrate levels are matching your needs. In other words, if you're eating enough carbohydrates to fuel your daily activity overall, then you'll be fine. Timing is a lower priority to quantity.

Protein: The intuitive idea is that eating protein after an intense workout prevents muscle breakdown and stimulates muscle protein synthesis (the incorporation of amino acids into skeletal muscle), resulting in increased muscle mass. That's certainly what I thought for many years, and still practice, even though I know the science doesn't exactly agree with this idea.

One study has shown that ingesting a relatively high amount of protein (40g rather 20g) post-exercise results in a greater degree of muscle protein synthesis that lasts for a longer period of time.[9]

In general, however, just like carbohydrates, the timing of when you get your protein has less impact than the quantity you are getting. We covered this extensively in Chapter 6 – on a plant-based diet, depending on your performance expectations, your protein requirements might be quite high.

Fats: The dogma has always been that eating fat after a workout will slow your digestive system down leading to the poor absorption of nutrients. Research doesn't completely agree. One study on the effects of consuming whole milk compared to skim milk showed that the whole milk increased the utilization of amino acids for protein synthesis, which could influence muscle growth.[10] Others have shown the high fat meals don't interfere with glycogen resynthesis. Overall, fat doesn't seem to be detrimental, and may even provide some benefit.

THERE IS NO BEFORE OR AFTER

Depending on the nature of the activity you're involved in, the food you eat before your workout may still have an effect on your post-workout recovery. If you exercise for a short time, and you eat a big meal an hour or so before you start, then the nutrients from that meal will be providing your body with the materials it needs to recover. So, there is a blurring of the boundaries between pre- and post-workout nutrition.

If you are consistently training, your nutrition needs are ongoing too. Research suggests that the best strategy is to have regularly timed "doses" of protein throughout the day – the best results for stimulating muscle protein synthesis is 20g every 3 hours.[11] If your protein requirements are particularly high, you could make sure you are supplementing at this level with this rate of interval. For most people, a 20g "dose" of protein will be the equivalent of a well-balanced meal containing a good protein source.

HYDRATION

You've heard this before, but you can't hear it enough times: make sure you drink enough water before and after working out. You can only achieve your best results when your body is properly hydrated. Your sweat contains water and electrolytes, which you lose when exercising and must replenish afterwards.

HOW MUCH WATER SHOULD YOU DRINK?

Pre-activity: You don't need to pre-hydrate before exercise if you stay hydrated. It is best to drink 5ml to 7ml per kg of body weight at least four hours before exercising if you are inadequately hydrated or if you have not hydrated for more than 8 to 12 hours since your last intense workout. Also avoid alcohol before an activity as it can have a dehydrating effect – you might feel this the next morning as well!

During the activity: During exercise, your fluid intake should be equal to the amount of fluid you are losing through sweat. This will prevent any negative health outcomes or a drop in performance. If you sweat a lot and don't replace the lost fluid, your blood volume will decrease, your blood pressure will drop, and your heart rate will increase to compensate. Small sips while you exercise will help performance, and fluid intake must take into account heat and humidity which will cause fluid loss to increase. If you're participating in a long event, then replacing lost electrolytes will also be important, especially if the conditions are particularly hot or humid.

Post activity: If you're really serious about post-exercise hydration, an effective way to know how much fluid you should drink is to weigh yourself before you start and after you finish your exercise. Your fluid intake should be adjusted based on how much has been lost. Consume 1.5 liters of water per kilogram of body weight lost during the training session if you wish to recover more rapidly.

WHEN SHOULD YOU EAT IF YOU'RE NOT TRAINING?

What if your nutritional needs aren't completely linked to your training schedule? As we discussed in Chapter 2, performance doesn't have to be thought of solely in terms of athleticism. Even if the tasks you need to perform aren't based directly on maximal muscle output, the timing of your mealtimes will still make a difference to how well you perform them.

IMPORTANCE OF MEALTIMES

If your diet is bad, it is unlikely that it will lead to great health in the future or improve your ability to handle your daily tasks, whenever you eat it. It doesn't matter how perfectly you time what you're eating if it is a diet of processed foods or low-nutrient, high-calorie snacks. However, our bodies do digest things differently at different times of day, and there are daily fluctuations that are influenced by our circadian rhythm, which is a cycle that moderates our patterns of sleep and wakefulness over the course of a 24-hour period. It serves as the body's internal clock, and it primarily reacts to light conditions.

Although the circadian rhythm is responsible for our sleep, it also affects digestion, metabolic patterns and other functions in the body. If your circadian rhythm is disrupted through broken sleep, it can have serious repercussions and cause widespread health problems. There have been many studies that have looked at the effects of both shift work that continues through the night and travelling between time zones.

Both cause significant disruption to the circadian rhythm with the knock-on effect of an increase in the risk of developing metabolic disorders, like insulin resistance and obesity.[12]

As well as disrupting the sleep cycle, working night shifts often means you consume more calories, and consume them at a time when the body is not expecting them. This can further impact the circadian rhythm which itself is affected by the timing of meals. You can think of the circadian rhythm as a centralized clock that controls all sorts of processes, like energy expenditure or the insulin sensitivity of the whole body. Peripheral clocks in organs or muscle groups help the regulation of this central clock – for instance, the peripheral clock in the gut regulates the absorption of glucose, the one in the pancreas regulates insulin secretion, the ones in major muscle groups regulate insulin sensitivity and so on. Eating at a time that is out of sync with your normal patterns means that there's a misalignment between these different clocks. The signals that regulate the central clock are being sent from the organs and muscles at conflicting times. This then affects how hormones are released and interact and can contribute to metabolic disorders.[13]

IS THERE A BEST TIME OF DAY TO EAT?

In simple terms, regular eating times are associated with an increase in energy and a reduction in the metabolic risk factors for chronic disease.[14] However, having this knowledge doesn't always make it easy to follow. When we eat can be influenced on a day-to-day basis by work, appetite, and social events, so it might not be possible for you to eat at the same time every day.

Here are some guidelines:

Breakfast: this meal literally breaks your overnight fast. There is some debate over the timing of this meal. People hold personal opinions on whether breakfast should be consumed as soon as they wake up versus waiting until later in the day when they have a larger appetite. Skipping breakfast seems to be a bad idea as studies have shown that this might make you prone to eating more calories at lunch and making less good meal choices throughout the rest of the day.[15] Eating more calories earlier on – for instance at breakfast – compared to later in the evening may help those who are trying to lose weight succeed in their efforts. Regularly skipping breakfast also appears to be correlated with a higher risk of death, specifically from cardiovascular disease.[16]

Lunch: just like breakfast, eating lunch earlier might help with weight loss efforts. Interesting research about the effect of meal timing on the microbiome has also shown that eating later can negatively affect its health and composition. The part of the microbiome that was examined was from the saliva and eating later increased the numbers of proinflammatory species of microbiota.[17] If your main meal of the day is going to be lunch, eating it earlier might lead to some positive health outcomes.

Dinner: the timing of this meal has the potential to have the biggest effect on long-term health. Melatonin is one of the main hormones that regulates the body's circadian rhythm as it controls your sleep cycle. It starts being produced when it first gets dark and gradually increases until it reaches a peak in the early hours of the morning. Increases in melatonin decrease the secretion of insulin which will mean the body will not metabolize sugars in the same way. Eating too close to the times when your body starts to release melatonin can therefore have a very negative effect on your health – obesity, metabolic syndrome and type 2 diabetes. Studies have also linked late night eating with dyslipidemia – elevated levels of fats in the blood, particularly "bad" LDL cholesterol – which can lead to cardiovascular disease.[18]

A QUICK FIX

You might have noticed that most of the advice surrounding food timing boils down to the same idea: *eat earlier in the day*.

One way of accomplishing this is to do a kind of intermittent fasting, where you only eat in a restricted window of time during the day. There are many different versions with different length windows, but studies have shown that restricting the total number of hours of eating to 12 or less will have a positive effect.[19] That means if you have breakfast at 8am, you need to have finished dinner before 8pm – and then strictly no snacking afterwards!

When I recommend intermittent fasting to my clients, by far the most effective has been a restricted window. There are other popular methods like 5-2 (five days eating normally, two days highly restricted), and these have had good effects on weight management, but I have found they can negatively impact performance. If you can cover your macronutrients in a 12-hour window, limiting your eating time can really improve your health.

CONCLUSION

There's no one single diet that's right for everyone, but hopefully by now you have all the available tools to create one that is right for you.

If you're thinking of adopting a plant-based diet, or you have already done so, it's a good idea to be clear in your mind as to why you're doing it. This will not only motivate you to stick with the diet, but also allow you to define how strict you are with it. For me, there has never been any question of switching back to eating animal products, and that has meant I've had to pay very close attention to my nutrition, making sure that I'm getting the macro and micronutrients that I need. If you follow a more flexitarian diet, it's much easier to cover your nutritional needs while getting a lot of the health benefits of eating more plants. Remember, research suggest that the more animal products you swap out for plants, the better the long-term health outcomes – whether that's from getting less animal fat and protein in your diet, eating more plants, or both.

Still, the level of performance you are expecting from your body will also determine how strict your nutritional plans need to be. High energy demands require sufficient calories, and heavy activity will also need a lot of protein to support recovery and growth. Optimizing your physical fitness means your nutrition must be optimized too. One of the biggest challenges facing those on a plant-based diet who are placing high physical demands on their body, is to get the right balance between protein-rich and high-fiber foods. You need to get the macronutrients in without getting too full. This can be really hard on a whole food diet, especially if you are engaged in heavy resistance training and have particularly high protein requirements.

There can be a large gap between creating the conditions inside your body to perform at your peak and having a dangerous nutrient deficiency. In other words, you might not be clinically deficient in some of the micronutrients that we covered in this book, but you might not be getting enough in an available format to be functioning at your best. Making sure you are getting everything you need takes some planning and calculation, but it is well worth putting in the time early on in your plant-based journey. The earlier you do it, the less likely you are to experience any adverse effects from lower than optimal levels of any micronutrients.

Likewise, if you take the time to take care of your gut health, the payoff in health terms is immeasurable. Your microbiome is part of what makes you unique. It contains its own genome that encodes countless proteins which are used in the body, and unlike the genome contained within your own cells, it is one that you can change. It is changed by what you eat, and by the decisions that you make every single day.

And that's the most important thing to remember. What you do matters. You can decide what food to eat, you can decide what impact you have on the world around you and the beings that live within it. Our greatest gift is our greatest responsibility: understanding the effects of our actions means that the actions we take must be responsible.

REFERENCES

Chapter 1

1 Redefine Meat (2021, Dec 15) *VEGAN STATISTICS – What is the Status in 2021?* https://www.redefinemeat.com/blog/vegan-statistics/

2 Statista (2021, Jan) *Value of the worldwide vegan food market from 2020 to 2021 with a forecast for 2025* https://www.statista.com/statistics/1280275/value-of-the-global-vegan-food-market/

3 Xu, X., Sharma, P., Shu, S. et al. Global greenhouse gas emissions from animal-based foods are twice those of plant-based foods. *Nat Food* 2, 724–732 (2021). https://doi.org/10.1038/s43016-021-00358-x

4 Aston LM, Smith JN, Powles JW (2012) Impact of a reduced red and processed meat dietary pattern on disease risks and greenhouse gas emissions in the UK: a modelling study, *BMJ Open* 2012;2:e001072. doi: 10.1136/bmjopen-2012-001072

5 E.M. Arrieta, A.D. González (2018), Impact of current, National Dietary Guidelines and alternative diets on greenhouse gas emissions in Argentina, *Food Policy*, Volume 79, 2018, Pages 58-66, ISSN 0306-9192, https://doi.org/10.1016/j.foodpol.2018.05.003.

6 Hertzler, S. R., Lieblein-Boff, J. C., Weiler, M., & Allgeier, C. (2020). Plant Proteins: Assessing Their Nutritional Quality and Effects on Health and Physical Function. *Nutrients*, *12*(12), 3704. https://doi.org/10.3390/nu12123704

7 Poore and T. Nemecek (2018), Reducing food's environmental impacts through producers and consumers, *Science* 360 (6392), 987-992, DOI: 10.1126/science.aaq0216o

8 Low P, Panksepp J, Reiss D, Edelman D, Van Swinderen B, Koch C (2012). "The Cambridge Declaration on Consciousness"

9 Animal Clock (2022) *2022 U.S. ANIMAL KILL CLOCK* https://animalclock.org/

10 Harish (2013, Mar 27) *Animals we use and abuse for food we do not eat.* Counting Animals. https://countinganimals.com/animals-we-use-and-abuse-for-food-we-do-not-eat/

11 Saunders, A. V., Davis, B. C., & Garg, M. L. (2013). Omega-3 polyunsaturated fatty acids and vegetarian diets. *The Medical journal of Australia*, 199(S4), S22–S26. https://doi.org/10.5694/mja11.11507

12 Kim, B., Hong, V. M., Yang, J., Hyun, H., Im, J. J., Hwang, J., Yoon, S., & Kim, J. E. (2016). A Review of Fermented Foods with Beneficial Effects on Brain and Cognitive Function. *Preventive nutrition and food science*, 21(4), 297–309. https://doi.org/10.3746/pnf.2016.21.4.297

13 Chen, X., Zhang, Z., Yang, H. et al. (2020) Consumption of ultra-processed foods and health outcomes: a systematic review of epidemiological studies. *Nutr J* 19, 86 https://doi.org/10.1186/s12937-020-00604-1

14 Srour, B., Fezeu, L., Kesse-Guyot, E., et. al. (2019) Ultra-processed food intake and risk of cardiovascular disease: prospective cohort study (NutriNet-Santé) *BMJ* 2019; 365 https://doi.org/10.1136/bmj.l1451

15 Rico-Campa, A., Martinez-Gonzalez, M., et. al., (2019), Association between consumption of ultra-processed foods and all cause mortality: SUN prospective cohort study, *BMJ* 2019; 365. https://doi.org/10.1136/bmj.l1949

16 Darmon, N., Darmon, M., Maillot, M., & Drewnowski, A. (2005). A nutrient density standard for vegetables and fruits: nutrients per calorie and nutrients per unit cost. *Journal of the American Dietetic Association*, *105*(12), 1881–1887. https://doi.org/10.1016/j.jada.2005.09.005

17 Di Noia J. Defining Powerhouse Fruits and Vegetables: A Nutrient Density

Approach. Prev Chronic Dis 2014;11:130390. DOI: http://dx.doi.org/10.5888/pcd11.130390

18 Stelmach-Mardas, M., Rodacki, T., Dobrowolska-Iwanek, J., Brzozowska, A., Walkowiak, J., Wojtanowska-Krosniak, A., Zagrodzki, P., Bechthold, A., Mardas, M., & Boeing, H. (2016). Link between Food Energy Density and Body Weight Changes in Obese Adults. *Nutrients*, 8(4), 229. https://doi.org/10.3390/nu8040229

19 McComb, S. E., & Mills, J. S. (2019). Orthorexia nervosa: A review of psychosocial risk factors. *Appetite*, 140, 50–75. https://doi.org/10.1016/j.appet.2019.05.005

Chapter 2

1 Kumar, A (2020, Apr 27) *The grandmaster diet: How to lose weight while barely moving.* ESPN. https://www.espn.co.uk/espn/story/_/id/27593253/why-grandmasters-magnus-carlsen-fabiano-caruana-lose-weight-playing-chess

2 Palacios C. (2006). The role of nutrients in bone health, from A to Z. *Critical reviews in food science and nutrition*, 46(8), 621–628. https://doi.org/10.1080/10408390500466174

3 Yang, Y., Yuan, Y., Tao, Y., & Wang, W. (2011). Effects of vitamin A deficiency on mucosal immunity and response to intestinal infection in rats. *Nutrition* (Burbank, Los Angeles County, Calif.), 27(2), 227–232. https://doi.org/10.1016/j.nut.2009.11.024

4 Thomas, J., Thomas, C. J., Radcliffe, J., & Itsiopoulos, C. (2015). Omega-3 Fatty Acids in Early Prevention of Inflammatory Neurodegenerative Disease: A Focus on Alzheimer's Disease. *BioMed research international*, 2015, 172801. https://doi.org/10.1155/2015/172801

5 Richardson A. J. (2006). Omega-3 fatty acids in ADHD and related neurodevelopmental disorders. *International review of psychiatry (Abingdon, England)*, 18(2), 155–172. https://doi.org/10.1080/09540260600583031

6 Wani, A. L., Bhat, S. A., & Ara, A. (2015). Omega-3 fatty acids and the treatment of depression: a review of scientific evidence. *Integrative medicine research*, 4(3), 132–141. https://doi.org/10.1016/j.imr.2015.07.003

7 Ljungberg, T., Bondza, E., & Lethin, C. (2020). Evidence of the Importance of Dietary Habits Regarding Depressive Symptoms and Depression. *International journal of environmental research and public health*, 17(5), 1616. https://doi.org/10.3390/ijerph17051616

8 Rao, T. S., Asha, M. R., Ramesh, B. N., & Rao, K. S. (2008). Understanding nutrition, depression and mental illnesses. *Indian journal of psychiatry*, 50(2), 77–82. https://doi.org/10.4103/0019-5545.42391

Chapter 3

1 Furman, D., Campisi, J., Verdin, E. et al. Chronic inflammation in the etiology of disease across the life span. *Nat Med* 25, 1822–1832 (2019). https://doi.org/10.1038/s41591-019-0675-0

2 Olfert, M. D., & Wattick, R. A. (2018). Vegetarian Diets and the Risk of Diabetes. *Current diabetes reports*, 18(11), 101. https://doi.org/10.1007/s11892-018-1070-9

3 McMacken, M., & Shah, S. (2017). A plant-based diet for the prevention and treatment of type 2 diabetes. *Journal of geriatric cardiology : JGC*, 14(5), 342–354. https://doi.org/10.11909/j.issn.1671-5411.2017.05.009

4 Tran, E., Dale, H. F., Jensen, C., & Lied, G. A. (2020). Effects of Plant-Based Diets on Weight Status: A Systematic Review. *Diabetes, metabolic syndrome and obesity : targets and therapy*, 13, 3433–3448. https://doi.org/10.2147/DMSO.S272802

5 Ryan, D. H., & Yockey, S. R. (2017). Weight Loss and Improvement in Comorbidity: Differences at 5%, 10%, 15%, and Over. *Current obesity reports*, 6(2), 187–194. https://doi.org/10.1007/s13679-017-0262-y

6 Kahleova, H., Fleeman, R., Hlozkova, A. *et al.* (2018). A plant-based diet in overweight individuals in a 16-week randomized clinical trial: metabolic benefits of plant protein. *Nutr & Diabetes* 8, 58 https://doi.org/10.1038/s41387-018-0067-4

7 Orlich, M. J., Singh, P. N., Sabaté, J., Jaceldo-Siegl, K., Fan, J., Knutsen, S., Beeson, W. L., & Fraser, G. E. (2013). Vegetarian dietary patterns and mortality in Adventist Health Study 2. *JAMA internal medicine*, 173(13), 1230–1238. https://doi.org/10.1001/jamainternmed.2013.6473

8 Tong, T., Appleby, P., Bradbury, K,. et al. (2019) Risks of ischaemic heart disease and stroke in meat eaters, fish eaters, and vegetarians over 18 years of follow-up: results from the prospective EPIC-Oxford study. *BMJ* 2019; 366 doi: https://doi.org/10.1136/bmj.l4897

9 Song, M., Fung, T. T., Hu, F. B., Willett, W. C., Longo, V. D., Chan, A. T., & Giovannucci, E. L. (2016). Association of Animal and Plant Protein Intake With All-Cause and Cause-Specific Mortality. *JAMA internal medicine*, 176(10), 1453–1463. https://doi.org/10.1001/jamainternmed.2016.4182

10 Barnard, N. D., Levin, S., Crosby, L., Flores, R., Holubkov, R., & Kahleova, H. (2022). A Randomized, Crossover Trial of a Nutritional Intervention for Rheumatoid Arthritis. *American Journal of Lifestyle Medicine.* https://doi.org/10.1177/15598276221081819

11 Masson, G., & Lamarche, B. (2016). Many non-elite multisport endurance athletes do not meet sports nutrition recommendations for carbohydrates. *Applied physiology, nutrition, and metabolism = Physiologie appliquee, nutrition et metabolisme*, 41(7), 728–734. https://doi.org/10.1139/apnm-2015-0599

12 Barnard, N. D., Goldman, D. M., Loomis, J. F., Kahleova, H., Levin, S. M., Neabore, S., & Batts, T. C. (2019). Plant-Based Diets for Cardiovascular Safety and Performance in Endurance Sports. *Nutrients*, 11(1), 130. https://doi.org/10.3390/nu11010130

13 van der Avoort, C., Jonvik, K. L., Nyakayiru, J., van Loon, L., Hopman, M., & Verdijk, L. B. (2020). A Nitrate-Rich Vegetable Intervention Elevates Plasma Nitrate and Nitrite Concentrations and Reduces Blood Pressure in Healthy Young Adults. *Journal of the Academy of Nutrition and Dietetics*, 120(8), 1305–1317. https://doi.org/10.1016/j.jand.2020.02.014

14 Szabo, Zoltan, Viktor Koczka, Tamas Marosvolgyi, Eva Szabo, Eszter Frank, Eva Polyak, Kata Fekete, Attila Erdelyi, Zsofia Verzar, and Maria Figler. (2021). Possible Biochemical Processes Underlying the Positive Health Effects of Plant-Based Diets—A Narrative Review *Nutrients* 13, no. 8: 2593. https://doi.org/10.3390/nu13082593

15 Beavers, K. M., Brinkley, T. E., & Nicklas, B. J. (2010). Effect of exercise training on chronic inflammation. Clinica chimica acta; international journal of clinical chemistry, 411(11-12), 785–793. https://doi.org/10.1016/j.cca.2010.02.069

16 Haghighatdoost, F., Bellissimo, N., Totosy de Zepetnek, J. O., & Rouhani, M. H. (2017). Association of vegetarian diet with inflammatory biomarkers: a systematic review and meta-analysis of observational studies. *Public health nutrition*, 20(15), 2713–2721. https://doi.org/10.1017/S1368980017001768

17 Segal, E., Elinav, E. (2017) *The Personalized Diet: The revolutionary plan to help you lose weight, prevent disease and feel incredible*

Chapter 4

1 Desmond, M. A., Sobiecki, J., Fewtrell, M., & Wells, J. (2018). Plant-based diets for children as a means of improving adult cardiometabolic health. *Nutrition reviews*, 76(4),

260–273. https://doi.org/10.1093/nutrit/nux079

2 Lan, T., Park, Y., Colditz, G. A., Liu, J., Wang, M., Wu, K., Giovannucci, E., & Sutcliffe, S. (2020). Adolescent dairy product and calcium intake in relation to later prostate cancer risk and mortality in the NIH-AARP Diet and Health Study. *Cancer causes & control : CCC*, 31(10), 891–904. https://doi.org/10.1007/s10552-020-01330-z

3 Tuso, P. J., Ismail, M. H., Ha, B. P., & Bartolotto, C. (2013). Nutritional update for physicians: plant-based diets. *The Permanente journal*, 17(2), 61–66. https://doi.org/10.7812/TPP/12-085

4 Weder, S., Hoffmann, M., Becker, K., Alexy, U., & Keller, M. (2019). Energy, Macronutrient Intake, and Anthropometrics of Vegetarian, Vegan, and Omnivorous Children (1¯3 Years) in Germany (VeChi Diet Study). *Nutrients*, 11(4), 832. https://doi.org/10.3390/nu11040832

Chapter 5

1 Clarys, P., Deliens, T., Huybrechts, I., Deriemaeker, P., Vanaelst, B., De Keyzer, W., Hebbelinck, M., & Mullie, P. (2014). Comparison of nutritional quality of the vegan, vegetarian, semi-vegetarian, pesco-vegetarian and omnivorous diet. *Nutrients*, 6(3), 1318–1332. https://doi.org/10.3390/nu6031318

2 Sabounchi, N. S., Rahmandad, H., & Ammerman, A. (2013). Best-fitting prediction equations for basal metabolic rate: informing obesity interventions in diverse populations. *International journal of obesity (2005)*, 37(10), 1364–1370. https://doi.org/10.1038/ijo.2012.218

3 M D Mifflin, S T St Jeor, L A Hill, B J Scott, S A Daugherty, Y O Koh, (1990) A new predictive equation for resting energy expenditure in healthy individuals, *The American Journal of Clinical Nutrition*, Volume 51, Issue 2, February 1990, Pages 241–247, https://doi.org/10.1093/ajcn/51.2.241

4 Food and Agriculture Organization of the United Nations. (2004). Human energy requirements: Energy Requirement of Adults. *Report of a Joint FAO/WHO/UNU Expert Consultation.*

5 Strasser, B., Spreitzer, A., & Haber, P. (2007). Fat loss depends on energy deficit only, independently of the method for weight loss. *Annals of nutrition & metabolism*, 51(5), 428–432. https://doi.org/10.1159/000111162

6 Benton, D., & Young, H. A. (2017). Reducing Calorie Intake May Not Help You Lose Body Weight. *Perspectives on psychological science : a journal of the Association for Psychological Science*, 12(5), 703–714. https://doi.org/10.1177/1745691617690878

7 Calcagno, M., Kahleova, H., Alwarith, J., Burgess, N. N., Flores, R. A., Busta, M. L., & Barnard, N. D. (2019). The Thermic Effect of Food: A Review. *Journal of the American College of Nutrition*, 38(6), 547–551. https://doi.org/10.1080/07315724.2018.1552544

8 Clark, M. J., & Slavin, J. L. (2013). The effect of fiber on satiety and food intake: a systematic review. *Journal of the American College of Nutrition*, 32(3), 200–211. https://doi.org/10.1080/07315724.2013.791194

9 Teff, K. L., Elliott, S. S., Tschöp, M., Kieffer, T. J., Rader, D., Heiman, M., Townsend, R. R., Keim, N. L., D'Alessio, D., & Havel, P. J. (2004). Dietary fructose reduces circulating insulin and leptin, attenuates postprandial suppression of ghrelin, and increases triglycerides in women. *The Journal of clinical endocrinology and metabolism*, 89(6), 2963–2972. https://doi.org/10.1210/jc.2003-031855

10 Wishnofsky, M., (1958) Caloric equivalents of gained or lost weight. *Am J Clin Nutr.* 1958; 6: 542-546

11 Thomas, D. M., Martin, C. K., Lettieri, S., Bredlau, C., Kaiser, K., Church, T., Bouchard, C., & Heymsfield, S. B. (2013). Can a weight loss of one pound a week be achieved with a 3500-kcal deficit? Commentary on a commonly accepted rule. *International journal of obesity (2005)*, 37(12), 1611–1613. https://doi.org/10.1038/ijo.2013.51

12 Rosenbaum, M., Vandenborne, K., Goldsmith, R., Simoneau, J. A., Heymsfield, S., Joanisse, D. R., Hirsch, J., Murphy, E., Matthews, D., Segal, K. R., & Leibel, R. L. (2003). Effects of experimental weight perturbation on skeletal muscle work efficiency in human subjects. *American journal of physiology. Regulatory, integrative and comparative physiology*, 285(1), R183–R192. https://doi.org/10.1152/ajpregu.00474.2002

13 Rosenbaum, M., & Leibel, R. L. (2010). Adaptive thermogenesis in humans. *International journal of obesity* (2005), 34 Suppl 1(0 1), S47–S55. https://doi.org/10.1038/ijo.2010.184

14 Heymsfield, S. B., Harp, J. B., Reitman, M. L., Beetsch, J. W., Schoeller, D. A., Erondu, N., & Pietrobelli, A. (2007). Why do obese patients not lose more weight when treated with low-calorie diets? A mechanistic perspective. *The American journal of clinical nutrition*, 85(2), 346–354. https://doi.org/10.1093/ajcn/85.2.346

15 U.S. Department of Agriculture and U.S. Department of Health and Human Services. *Dietary Guidelines for Americans, 2020-2025*. 9th Edition. December 2020. Available at DietaryGuidelines.gov

16 Institute of Medicine. Dietary carbohydrates, sugars and starches. In: *Dietary Reference Intakes for Energy, Carbohydrates, Fiber, Fat, Fatty Acids, Cholesterol, Protein, and Amino Acids*. Washington, DC: National Academies Press; 2005:265–338.

17 Slavin, J., & Carlson, J. (2014). Carbohydrates. *Advances in nutrition* (Bethesda, Md.), 5(6), 760–761. https://doi.org/10.3945/an.114.006163

18 Kerksick, C. M., Arent, S., Schoenfeld, B. J., Stout, J. R., Campbell, B., Wilborn, C. D., Taylor, L., Kalman, D., Smith-Ryan, A. E., Kreider, R. B., Willoughby, D., Arciero, P. J., VanDusseldorp, T. A., Ormsbee, M. J., Wildman, R., Greenwood, M., Ziegenfuss, T. N., Aragon, A. A., & Antonio, J. (2017). International society of sports nutrition position stand: nutrient timing. *Journal of the International Society of Sports Nutrition*, 14, 33. https://doi.org/10.1186/s12970-017-0189-4

19 Veit, M., van Asten, R., Olie, A. et al. (2022) The role of dietary sugars, overweight, and obesity in type 2 diabetes mellitus: a narrative review. *Eur J Clin Nutr* https://doi.org/10.1038/s41430-022-01114-5

20 Chandler-Laney, P. C., Morrison, S. A., Goree, L. L., Ellis, A. C., Casazza, K., Desmond, R., & Gower, B. A. (2014). Return of hunger following a relatively high carbohydrate breakfast is associated with earlier recorded glucose peak and nadir. *Appetite*, 80, 236–241. https://doi.org/10.1016/j.appet.2014.04.031

21 Bray G. A. (2013). Energy and fructose from beverages sweetened with sugar or high-fructose corn syrup pose a health risk for some people. *Advances in nutrition* (Bethesda, Md.), 4(2), 220–225. https://doi.org/10.3945/an.112.002816

22 Schulze, M. B., Manson, J. E., Ludwig, D. S., Colditz, G. A., Stampfer, M. J., Willett, W. C., & Hu, F. B. (2004). Sugar-sweetened beverages, weight gain, and incidence of type 2 diabetes in young and middle-aged women. *JAMA*, 292(8), 927–934. https://doi.org/10.1001/jama.292.8.927

23 Alizadeh, M., Gharaaghaji, R., & Gargari, B. P. (2014). The effects of legumes on metabolic features, insulin resistance and hepatic function tests in women with central obesity: a randomized controlled trial. *International journal of preventive medicine*, 5(6), 710–720.

24 Afshin, A., Micha, R., Khatibzadeh, S., & Mozaffarian, D. (2014). Consumption of nuts and legumes and risk of incident ischemic heart disease, stroke, and diabetes: a systematic review and meta-analysis. *The American journal of clinical nutrition*, 100(1), 278–288. https://doi.org/10.3945/ajcn.113.076901

25 Wu, H., Flint, A. J., Qi, Q., van Dam, R. M., Sampson, L. A., Rimm, E. B., Holmes, M. D., Willett, W. C., Hu, F. B., & Sun, Q. (2015). Association between dietary whole grain intake and risk of mortality: two large prospective studies in US men and women. *JAMA internal medicine*, 175(3), 373–384. https://doi.org/10.1001/jamainternmed.2014.6283

26 Greenwood, D. C., Threapleton, D. E., Evans, C. E., Cleghorn, C. L., Nykjaer, C., Woodhead, C., & Burley, V. J. (2013). Glycemic index, glycemic load, carbohydrates, and type 2 diabetes: systematic review and dose-response meta-analysis of prospective studies. *Diabetes care, 36*(12), 4166–4171. https://doi.org/10.2337/dc13-0325
27 Howarth, N. C., Saltzman, E., & Roberts, S. B. (2001). Dietary fiber and weight regulation. *Nutrition reviews, 59*(5), 129–139. https://doi.org/10.1111/j.1753-4887.2001.tb07001.x

Chapter 6

1 Li, P., Yin, Y. L., Li, D., Kim, S. W., & Wu, G. (2007). Amino acids and immune function. *The British journal of nutrition, 98*(2), 237–252. https://doi.org/10.1017/S000711450769936X
2 MacKenzie, E. L., Iwasaki, K., & Tsuji, Y. (2008). Intracellular iron transport and storage: from molecular mechanisms to health implications. *Antioxidants & redox signaling, 10*(6), 997–1030. https://doi.org/10.1089/ars.2007.1893
3 Wu G. (2016). Dietary protein intake and human health. *Food & function, 7*(3), 1251–1265. https://doi.org/10.1039/c5fo01530h
4 Lemon P. W. (1995). Do athletes need more dietary protein and amino acids?. *International journal of sport nutrition, 5 Suppl*, S39–S61. https://doi.org/10.1123/ijsn.5.s1.s39
5 Campbell, B., Kreider, R. B., Ziegenfuss, T., La Bounty, P., Roberts, M., Burke, D., Landis, J., Lopez, H., & Antonio, J. (2007). International Society of Sports Nutrition position stand: protein and exercise. *Journal of the International Society of Sports Nutrition, 4*, 8. https://doi.org/10.1186/1550-2783-4-8
6 Stokes, T., Hector, A. J., Morton, R. W., McGlory, C., & Phillips, S. M. (2018). Recent Perspectives Regarding the Role of Dietary Protein for the Promotion of Muscle Hypertrophy with Resistance Exercise Training. *Nutrients, 10*(2), 180. https://doi.org/10.3390/nu10020180
7 Morton, R. W., Murphy, K. T., McKellar, S. R., Schoenfeld, B. J., Henselmans, M., Helms, E., Aragon, A. A., Devries, M. C., Banfield, L., Krieger, J. W., & Phillips, S. M. (2018). A systematic review, meta-analysis and meta-regression of the effect of protein supplementation on resistance training-induced gains in muscle mass and strength in healthy adults. *British journal of sports medicine, 52*(6), 376–384. https://doi.org/10.1136/bjsports-2017-097608
8 Becerra-Tomás, N., Díaz-López, A., Rosique-Esteban, N., Ros, E., Buil-Cosiales, P., Corella, D., Estruch, R., Fitó, M., Serra-Majem, L., Arós, F., Lamuela-Raventós, R. M., Fiol, M., Santos-Lozano, J. M., Díez-Espino, J., Portoles, O., Salas-Salvadó, J., & PREDIMED Study Investigators (2018). Legume consumption is inversely associated with type 2 diabetes incidence in adults: A prospective assessment from the PREDIMED study. *Clinical nutrition* (Edinburgh, Scotland), 37(3), 906–913. https://doi.org/10.1016/j.clnu.2017.03.015
9 Key, T. (2011). Diet, insulin-like growth factor-1 and cancer risk. *Proceedings of the Nutrition Society, 70*(3), 385-388. doi:10.1017/S0029665111000127
10 Levey, A. S., Adler, S., Caggiula, A. W., England, B. K., Greene, T., Hunsicker, L. G., Kusek, J. W., Rogers, N. L., & Teschan, P. E. (1996). Effects of dietary protein restriction on the progression of advanced renal disease in the Modification of Diet in Renal Disease Study. *American journal of kidney diseases : the official journal of the National Kidney Foundation, 27*(5), 652–663. https://doi.org/10.1016/s0272-6386(96)90099-2
11 Chen, X., Wei, G., Jalili, T., Metos, J., Giri, A., Cho, M. E., Boucher, R., Greene, T., & Beddhu, S. (2016). The Associations of Plant Protein Intake With All-Cause Mortality in CKD. *American journal of kidney diseases : the official journal of the National Kidney*

Foundation, 67(3), 423–430. https://doi.org/10.1053/j.ajkd.2015.10.018

12 Hernández-Alonso, P., Salas-Salvadó, J., Ruiz-Canela, M., et al. (2015). High dietary protein intake is associated with an increased body weight and total death risk. *Clinical Nutrition*, Volume 35, Issue 2, P496-506, April 01, 2016. https://doi.org/10.1016/j.clnu.2015.03.016

13 Hamilton-Reeves, J. M., Vazquez, G., Duval, S. J., Phipps, W. R., Kurzer, M. S., & Messina, M. J. (2010). Clinical studies show no effects of soy protein or isoflavones on reproductive hormones in men: results of a meta-analysis. *Fertility and sterility*, 94(3), 997–1007. https://doi.org/10.1016/j.fertnstert.2009.04.038

14 Sathyapalan T, Dawson AJ, Rigby AS, Thatcher NJ, Kilpatrick ES, Atkin SL. The Effect of Phytoestrogen on Thyroid in Subclinical Hypothyroidism: Randomized, Double Blind, Crossover Study. *Front Endocrinol* (Lausanne). 2018 Sep 11;9:531. doi: 10.3389/fendo.2018.00531. PMID: 30254609; PMCID: PMC6141627.

15 Meftaul, I. M., Venkateswarlu, K., Dharmarajan, R., Annamalai, P., Asaduzzaman, M., Parven, A., & Megharaj, M. (2020). Controversies over human health and ecological impacts of glyphosate: Is it to be banned in modern agriculture?. *Environmental pollution* (Barking, Essex : 1987), 263(Pt A), 114372. https://doi.org/10.1016/j.envpol.2020.114372

Chapter 7

1 Volek, J. S., Kraemer, W. J., Bush, J. A., Incledon, T., & Boetes, M. (1997). Testosterone and cortisol in relationship to dietary nutrients and resistance exercise. *Journal of applied physiology* (Bethesda, Md. : 1985), 82(1), 49–54. https://doi.org/10.1152/jappl.1997.82.1.49

2 Zhong VW, Van Horn L, Cornelis MC, et al. Associations of Dietary Cholesterol or Egg Consumption With Incident Cardiovascular Disease and Mortality. *JAMA*. 2019;321(11):1081–1095. doi:10.1001/jama.2019.1572

3 Siri-Tarino, P. W., Sun, Q., Hu, F. B., & Krauss, R. M. (2010). Saturated fatty acids and risk of coronary heart disease: modulation by replacement nutrients. *Current atherosclerosis reports*, 12(6), 384–390. https://doi.org/10.1007/s11883-010-0131-6

4 American Heart Associaton (2021, Nov 1) *Saturated Fat* https://www.heart.org/en/healthy-living/healthy-eating/eat-smart/fats/saturated-fats

5 Brouwer, I. A., Wanders, A. J., & Katan, M. B. (2010). Effect of animal and industrial trans fatty acids on HDL and LDL cholesterol levels in humans--a quantitative review. *PloS one*, 5(3), e9434. https://doi.org/10.1371/journal.pone.0009434

6 Schwingshackl, L., & Hoffmann, G. (2012). Monounsaturated fatty acids and risk of cardiovascular disease: synopsis of the evidence available from systematic reviews and meta-analyses. *Nutrients*, 4(12), 1989–2007. https://doi.org/10.3390/nu4121989

7 Ander, B. P., Dupasquier, C. M., Prociuk, M. A., & Pierce, G. N. (2003). Polyunsaturated fatty acids and their effects on cardiovascular disease. *Experimental and clinical cardiology*, 8(4), 164–172.

8 Vogel, R. A., Corretti, M. C., & Plotnick, G. D. (1997). Effect of a single high-fat meal on endothelial function in healthy subjects. *The American journal of cardiology*, 79(3), 350–354. https://doi.org/10.1016/s0002-9149(96)00760-6

9 Henning, A. L., Venable, A. S., Vingren, J. L., Hill, D. W., & McFarlin, B. K. (2018). Consumption of a high-fat meal was associated with an increase in monocyte adhesion molecules, scavenger receptors, and Propensity to Form Foam Cells. Cytometry. Part B, *Clinical cytometry*, 94(4), 606–612. https://doi.org/10.1002/cyto.b.21478

10 Neale, E. P., Tapsell, L. C., Guan, V. & Batterham, M. J. (2017). The effect of nut consumption on markers of inflammation and endothelial function: A systematic review and meta-analysis of randomised controlled trials. *BMJ Open*, 7 (11), e016863-1-e016863-14.

11 Patterson, E., Wall, R., Fitzgerald, G. F., Ross, R. P., & Stanton, C. (2012). Health implications of high dietary omega-6 polyunsaturated Fatty acids. *Journal of nutrition and metabolism*, 2012, 539426. https://doi.org/10.1155/2012/539426

12 Hibbeln, J. R., Nieminen, L. R., Blasbalg, T. L., Riggs, J. A., & Lands, W. E. (2006). Healthy intakes of n-3 and n-6 fatty acids: estimations considering worldwide diversity. *The American journal of clinical nutrition*, 83(6 Suppl), 1483S–1493S. https://doi.org/10.1093/ajcn/83.6.1483S

13 Harris, W. S., Mozaffarian, D., Rimm, E., Kris-Etherton, P., Rudel, L. L., Appel, L. J., Engler, M. M., Engler, M. B., & Sacks, F. (2009). Omega-6 fatty acids and risk for cardiovascular disease: a science advisory from the American Heart Association Nutrition Subcommittee of the Council on Nutrition, Physical Activity, and Metabolism; Council on Cardiovascular Nursing; and Council on Epidemiology and Prevention. *Circulation*, 119(6), 902–907. https://doi.org/10.1161/CIRCULATIONAHA.108.191627

14 O'keefe, S., Gaskins-wright, S., Wiley, V. And CHEN, I.-C. (1994), Levels Of Trans Geometrical Isomers Of Essential Fatty Acids In Some Unhydrogenated U. S. Vegetable Oils. *Journal of Food Lipids*, 1: 165-176. https://doi.org/10.1111/j.1745-4522.1994.tb00244.x

15 Bhardwaj, S., Passi, S. J., Misra, A., Pant, K. K., Anwar, K., Pandey, R. M., & Kardam, V. (2016). Effect of heating/reheating of fats/oils, as used by Asian Indians, on trans fatty acid formation. *Food chemistry*, 212, 663–670. https://doi.org/10.1016/j.foodchem.2016.06.021

16 Santos, F. L., Esteves, S. S., da Costa Pereira, A., Yancy, W. S., Jr, & Nunes, J. P. (2012). Systematic review and meta-analysis of clinical trials of the effects of low carbohydrate diets on cardiovascular risk factors. *Obesity reviews : an official journal of the International Association for the Study of Obesity*, 13(11), 1048–1066. https://doi.org/10.1111/j.1467-789X.2012.01021.x

17 Bailey, C.P., Hennessy, E. A review of the ketogenic diet for endurance athletes: performance enhancer or placebo effect?. *J Int Soc Sports Nutr* **17**, 33 (2020). https://doi.org/10.1186/s12970-020-00362-9

Chapter 8

1 de Benoist, B., McLean, E., Egli, I., Cogswell, M. (2005) Worldwide prevalence of anaemia 1993–2005 : WHO global database on anaemia

2 Herrmann, W., Schorr, H., Obeid, R., & Geisel, J. (2003). Vitamin B-12 status, particularly holotranscobalamin II and methylmalonic acid concentrations, and hyperhomocysteinemia in vegetarians. *The American journal of clinical nutrition*, 78(1), 131–136. https://doi.org/10.1093/ajcn/78.1.131

3 Rizzo G, Laganà AS, Rapisarda AM, La Ferrera GM, Buscema M, Rossetti P, Nigro A, Muscia V, Valenti G, Sapia F, Sarpietro G, Zigarelli M, Vitale SG. Vitamin B12 among Vegetarians: Status, Assessment and Supplementation. *Nutrients*. 2016 Nov 29;8(12):767. doi: 10.3390/nu8120767. PMID: 27916823; PMCID: PMC5188422.

4 Smith, A. D., Refsum, H., Bottiglieri, T., Fenech, M., Hooshmand, B., McCaddon, A., Miller, J. W., Rosenberg, I. H., & Obeid, R. (2018). Homocysteine and Dementia: An International Consensus Statement. *Journal of Alzheimer's disease : JAD*, 62(2), 561–570. https://doi.org/10.3233/JAD-171042

5 Institute of Medicine (US) Standing Committee on the Scientific Evaluation of Dietary Reference Intakes and its Panel on Folate, Other B Vitamins, and Choline. Dietary Reference Intakes for Thiamin, Riboflavin, Niacin, Vitamin B6, Folate, Vitamin B12, Pantothenic Acid, Biotin, and Choline. Washington (DC): National Academies Press (US); 1998. N, Estimation of the Period Covered by Vitamin B12 Stores. Available from: https://www.ncbi.nlm.nih.gov/books/NBK114329/

6 Smith, A. D., Warren, M. J., & Refsum, H. (2018). Vitamin B12. *Advances in food and nutrition research*, 83, 215–279. https://doi.org/10.1016/bs.afnr.2017.11.005

7 Deshmukh, U. S., Joglekar, C. V., Lubree, H. G., Ramdas, L. V., Bhat, D. S., Naik, S. S., Hardikar, P. S., Raut, D. A., Konde, T. B., Wills, A. K., Jackson, A. A., Refsum, H., Nanivadekar, A. S., Fall, C. H., & Yajnik, C. S. (2010). Effect of physiological doses of oral vitamin B12 on plasma homocysteine: a randomized, placebo-controlled, double-blind trial in India. *European journal of clinical nutrition*, 64(5), 495–502. https://doi.org/10.1038/ejcn.2010.15

8 Del Bo', C., Riso, P., Gardana, C., Brusamolino, A., Battezzati, A., & Ciappellano, S. (2019). Effect of two different sublingual dosages of vitamin B12 on cobalamin nutritional status in vegans and vegetarians with a marginal deficiency: A randomized controlled trial. *Clinical nutrition* (Edinburgh, Scotland), 38(2), 575–583. https://doi.org/10.1016/j.clnu.2018.02.008

9 Thakkar, K., & Billa, G. (2015). Treatment of vitamin B12 deficiency-methylcobalamine? Cyancobalamine? Hydroxocobalamin?-clearing the confusion. *European journal of clinical nutrition*, 69(1), 1–2. https://doi.org/10.1038/ejcn.2014.165

10 Vegan Health (2022, May) *Vitamin B12: Rationale for VeganHealth's Recommendations* https://veganhealth.org/vitamin-b12/explanation-of-vitamin-b12-recommendations/

11 Davis, B. & Kris-Etherton, P. (2003). Achieving optimal essential fatty acid status in vegetarians: current knowledge and practical implications, *The American Journal of Clinical Nutrition*, Volume 78, Issue 3, September 2003, Pages 640S–646S, https://doi.org/10.1093/ajcn/78.3.640S

12 Anderson, B. M., & Ma, D. W. (2009). Are all n-3 polyunsaturated fatty acids created equal?. *Lipids in health and disease*, 8, 33. https://doi.org/10.1186/1476-511X-8-33

13 U.S. Department of Agriculture and U.S. Department of Health and Human Services. *Dietary Guidelines for Americans, 2020-2025.* 9th Edition. December 2020. Available at DietaryGuidelines.gov

14 Dobnig H. (2011). A review of the health consequences of the vitamin D deficiency pandemic. *Journal of the neurological sciences*, 311(1-2), 15–18. https://doi.org/10.1016/j.jns.2011.08.046

15 Chowdhury, R., Kunutsor, S., Vitezova, A., Oliver-Williams, C., Chowdhury, S., Kiefte-de-Jong, J. C., Khan, H., Baena, C. P., Prabhakaran, D., Hoshen, M. B., Feldman, B. S., Pan, A., Johnson, L., Crowe, F., Hu, F. B., & Franco, O. H. (2014). Vitamin D and risk of cause specific death: systematic review and meta-analysis of observational cohort and randomised intervention studies. *BMJ* (Clinical research ed.), 348, g1903. https://doi.org/10.1136/bmj.g1903

16 Ambroszkiewicz, J., Klemarczyk, W., Gajewska, J., Chełchowska, M., Franek, E., & Laskowska-Klita, T. (2010). The influence of vegan diet on bone mineral density and biochemical bone turnover markers. *Pediatric endocrinology, diabetes, and metabolism*, 16(3), 201–204.

17 Tomlinson, P. B., Joseph, C., & Angioi, M. (2015). Effects of vitamin D supplementation on upper and lower body muscle strength levels in healthy individuals. A systematic review with meta-analysis. *Journal of science and medicine in sport*, 18(5), 575–580. https://doi.org/10.1016/j.jsams.2014.07.022

18 Institute of Medicine (US) Standing Committee on the Scientific Evaluation of Dietary Reference Intakes. Dietary Reference Intakes for Calcium, Phosphorus, Magnesium, Vitamin D, and Fluoride. Washington (DC): National Academies Press (US); 1997. 1, Dietary Reference Intakes. Available from: https://www.ncbi.nlm.nih.gov/books/NBK109829/

19 Zeisel, S. H., & da Costa, K. A. (2009). Choline: an essential nutrient for public

health. *Nutrition reviews, 67*(11), 615–623. https://doi.org/10.1111/
j.1753-4887.2009.00246.x

20 Subramaniam, G., & Girish, M. (2015). Iron deficiency anemia in children. *Indian journal of pediatrics, 82*(6), 558–564. https://doi.org/10.1007/s12098-014-1643-9

21 Pawlak R, Berger J, Hines I. Iron Status of Vegetarian Adults: A Review of Literature. Am J Lifestyle Med. 2016 Dec 16;12(6):486-498. doi: 10.1177/1559827616682933. PMID: 30783404; PMCID: PMC6367879.

22 Ma, Q., Kim, E. Y., Lindsay, E. A., & Han, O. (2011). Bioactive dietary polyphenols inhibit heme iron absorption in a dose-dependent manner in human intestinal Caco-2 cells. *Journal of food science, 76*(5), H143–H150. https://doi.org/10.1111/
j.1750-3841.2011.02184.x

23 Compoundchem (2018, July 17) *The chemistry of spinach: the iron myth and 'spinach teeth'* https://www.compoundchem.com/2018/07/17/spinach/

24 Trumbo, P., Yates, A. A., Schlicker, S., & Poos, M. (2001). Dietary reference intakes: vitamin A, vitamin K, arsenic, boron, chromium, copper, iodine, iron, manganese, molybdenum, nickel, silicon, vanadium, and zinc. *Journal of the American Dietetic Association, 101*(3), 294–301. https://doi.org/10.1016/S0002-8223(01)00078-5

25 Lukaski H. C. (2004). Vitamin and mineral status: effects on physical performance. *Nutrition (Burbank, Los Angeles County, Calif.), 20*(7-8), 632–644. https://doi.org/10.1016/j.nut.2004.04.001

26 Thomas, D. T., Erdman, K. A., & Burke, L. M. (2016). American College of Sports Medicine Joint Position Statement. Nutrition and Athletic Performance. *Medicine and science in sports and exercise, 48*(3), 543–568. https://doi.org/10.1249/
MSS.0000000000000852

27 Fang, A., Li, K., Li, H. *et al.* Low Habitual Dietary Calcium and Linear Growth from Adolescence to Young Adulthood: results from the China Health and Nutrition Survey. *Sci Rep* 7, 9111 (2017). https://doi.org/10.1038/s41598-017-08943-6

28 Warensjö, E., Byberg, L., Melhus, H., Gedeborg, R., Mallmin, H., Wolk, A., & Michaëlsson, K. (2011). Dietary calcium intake and risk of fracture and osteoporosis: prospective longitudinal cohort study. *BMJ* (Clinical research ed.), 342, d1473. https://doi.org/10.1136/bmj.d1473

29 Ho-Pham, L. T., Nguyen, N. D., & Nguyen, T. V. (2009). Effect of vegetarian diets on bone mineral density: a Bayesian meta-analysis. *The American journal of clinical nutrition, 90*(4), 943–950. https://doi.org/10.3945/ajcn.2009.27521

30 Li, K., Wang, X. F., Li, D. Y., Chen, Y. C., Zhao, L. J., Liu, X. G., Guo, Y. F., Shen, J., Lin, X., Deng, J., Zhou, R., & Deng, H. W. (2018). The good, the bad, and the ugly of calcium supplementation: a review of calcium intake on human health. *Clinical interventions in aging, 13*, 2443–2452. https://doi.org/10.2147/CIA.S157523

31 Foster, M., Chu, A., Petocz, P., & Samman, S. (2013). Effect of vegetarian diets on zinc status: a systematic review and meta-analysis of studies in humans. *Journal of the science of food and agriculture, 93*(10), 2362–2371. https://doi.org/10.1002/jsfa.6179

32 Sobiecki, J. G., Appleby, P. N., Bradbury, K. E., & Key, T. J. (2016). High compliance with dietary recommendations in a cohort of meat eaters, fish eaters, vegetarians, and vegans: results from the European Prospective Investigation into Cancer and Nutrition-Oxford study. *Nutrition research* (New York, N.Y.), 36(5), 464–477. https://doi.org/
10.1016/j.nutres.2015.12.016\

33 National Academic Press (2001) *Dietary Reference Intakes for Vitamin A, Vitamin K, Arsenic, Boron, Chromium, Copper, Iodine, Iron, Manganese, Molybdenum, Nickel, Silicon, Vanadium, and Zinc* https://nap.nationalacademies.org/read/10026/chapter/14

34 Li, Y., Liu, K., Shen, J., & Liu, Y. (2016). Wheat bran intake can attenuate chronic cadmium toxicity in mice gut microbiota. *Food & function, 7*(8), 3524–3530. https://doi.org/10.1039/c6fo00233a

35 McCarty M. F. (2012). Zinc and multi-mineral supplementation should mitigate the pathogenic impact of cadmium exposure. *Medical hypotheses*, 79(5), 642–648. https://doi.org/10.1016/j.mehy.2012.07.043

36 Zimmermann, M. B., & Andersson, M. (2012). Assessment of iodine nutrition in populations: past, present, and future. *Nutrition reviews*, 70(10), 553–570. https://doi.org/10.1111/j.1753-4887.2012.00528.x

37 Weikert, C., Trefflich, I., Menzel, J., Obeid, R., Longree, A., Dierkes, J., Meyer, K., Herter-Aeberli, I., Mai, K., Stangl, G. I., Müller, S. M., Schwerdtle, T., Lampen, A., & Abraham, K. (2020). Vitamin and Mineral Status in a Vegan Diet. *Deutsches Arzteblatt international*, 117(35-36), 575–582. https://doi.org/10.3238/arztebl.2020.0575

Chapter 9

1 Kreider, R.B., Kalman, D.S., Antonio, J. *et al*. International Society of Sports Nutrition position stand: safety and efficacy of creatine supplementation in exercise, sport, and medicine. *J Int Soc Sports Nutr* 14, 18 (2017) https://doi.org/10.1186/s12970-017-0173-z

2 Burke, D. G., Chilibeck, P. D., Parise, G., Candow, D. G., Mahoney, D., & Tarnopolsky, M. (2003). Effect of creatine and weight training on muscle creatine and performance in vegetarians. *Medicine and science in sports and exercise*, 35(11), 1946–1955. https://doi.org/10.1249/01.MSS.0000093614.17517.79

3 Rae, C., Digney, A. L., McEwan, S. R., & Bates, T. C. (2003). Oral creatine monohydrate supplementation improves brain performance: a double-blind, placebo-controlled, cross-over trial. *Proceedings. Biological sciences*, 270(1529), 2147–2150. https://doi.org/10.1098/rspb.2003.2492

4 Kreider, R. B., Kalman, D. S., Antonio, J., Ziegenfuss, T. N., Wildman, R., Collins, R., Candow, D. G., Kleiner, S. M., Almada, A. L., & Lopez, H. L. (2017). International Society of Sports Nutrition position stand: safety and efficacy of creatine supplementation in exercise, sport, and medicine. *Journal of the International Society of Sports Nutrition*, 14, 18. https://doi.org/10.1186/s12970-017-0173-z

5 Pekala, J., Patkowska-Sokoła, B., Bodkowski, R., Jamroz, D., Nowakowski, P., Lochyński, S., & Librowski, T. (2011). L-carnitine--metabolic functions and meaning in humans life. *Current drug metabolism*, 12(7), 667–678. https://doi.org/10.2174/138920011796504536

6 Stephens, F. B., Marimuthu, K., Cheng, Y., Patel, N., Constantin, D., Simpson, E. J., & Greenhaff, P. L. (2011). Vegetarians have a reduced skeletal muscle carnitine transport capacity. *The American journal of clinical nutrition*, 94(3), 938–944. https://doi.org/10.3945/ajcn.111.012047

7 Cahova, M., Christina, P., Hansikova, H., et al. (2014). Carnitine supplementation alleviates lipid metabolism derangements and protects against oxidative stress in non-obese hereditary hypertriglyceridemic rats. *Applied Physiology, Nutrition, and Metabolism*. 40(3): 280-291. https://doi.org/10.1139/apnm-2014-0163

8 Kurtz JA, VanDusseldorp TA, Doyle JA, Otis JS. (2021) Taurine in sports and exercise. *J Int Soc Sports Nutr*. 2021 May 26;18(1):39. doi: 10.1186/s12970-021-00438-0. PMID: 34039357; PMCID: PMC8152067.

9 Wang, A. M., Ma, C., Xie, Z. H., & Shen, F. (2000). Use of carnosine as a natural anti-senescence drug for human beings. *Biochemistry. Biokhimiia*, 65(7), 869–871.

10 Varanoske, A. N., Hoffman, J. R., Church, D. D., Wang, R., Baker, K. M., Dodd, S. J., Coker, N. A., Oliveira, L. P., Dawson, V. L., Fukuda, D. H., & Stout, J. R. (2017). Influence of Skeletal Muscle Carnosine Content on Fatigue during Repeated Resistance Exercise in Recreationally Active Women. *Nutrients*, 9(9), 988. https://doi.org/10.3390/nu9090988

11 Trč, T., & Bohmová, J. (2011). Efficacy and tolerance of enzymatic hydrolysed collagen (EHC) vs. glucosamine sulphate (GS) in the treatment of knee osteoarthritis (KOA). *International orthopaedics*, 35(3), 341–348. https://doi.org/10.1007/s00264-010-1010-z

Chapter 10

1 Stinson, L., Boyce, M., Payne, M., Keelan, J., (2019). The Not-so-Sterile Womb: Evidence That the Human Fetus Is Exposed to Bacteria Prior to Birth. *Frontiers in Microbiology*, 04 June 2019. https://doi.org/10.3389/fmicb.2019.01124

2 Mosca, A., Leclerc, M., Hugot, J. (2016) Gut Microbiota Diversity and Human Diseases: Should We Reintroduce Key Predators in Our Ecosystem? *Frontiers in Microbiology* 31 March 2016 https://doi.org/10.3389/fmicb.2016.00455

3 Li, Y., Hao, Y., Fan, F., & Zhang, B. (2018). The Role of Microbiome in Insomnia, Circadian Disturbance and Depression. *Frontiers in psychiatry*, 9, 669. https://doi.org/10.3389/fpsyt.2018.00669

4 Stasi, C., Sadalla, S., & Milani, S. (2019). The Relationship Between the Serotonin Metabolism, Gut-Microbiota and the Gut-Brain Axis. Current drug metabolism, 20(8), 646–655. https://doi.org/10.2174/1389200220666190725115503

5 De Pessemier, B., Grine, L., Debaere, M., Maes, A., Paetzold, B., & Callewaert, C. (2021). Gut-Skin Axis: Current Knowledge of the Interrelationship between Microbial Dysbiosis and Skin Conditions. Microorganisms, 9(2), 353. https://doi.org/10.3390/microorganisms9020353

6 Vighi, G., Marcucci, F., Sensi, L., Di Cara, G., & Frati, F. (2008). Allergy and the gastrointestinal system. Clinical and experimental immunology, 153 Suppl 1(Suppl 1), 3–6. https://doi.org/10.1111/j.1365-2249.2008.03713.x

7 Wu, H. J., & Wu, E. (2012). The role of gut microbiota in immune homeostasis and autoimmunity. *Gut microbes*, 3(1), 4–14. https://doi.org/10.4161/gmic.19320

8 Corcoran, B. M., Stanton, C., Fitzgerald, G. F., & Ross, R. P. (2005). Survival of probiotic lactobacilli in acidic environments is enhanced in the presence of metabolizable sugars. *Applied and environmental microbiology*, 71(6), 3060–3067. https://doi.org/10.1128/AEM.71.6.3060-3067.2005

9 De Filippo, C., Cavalieri, D., Di Paola, M., et al. (2010). Impact of diet in shaping gut microbiota revealed by a comparative study in children from Europe and rural Africa. Proceedings of the National Academy of Sciences (PNAS). 107 (33) 14691-14696 https://doi.org/10.1073/pnas.100596310

10 Losasso, C., Eckert, E. M., Mastrorilli, E., Villiger, J., Mancin, M., Patuzzi, I., Di Cesare, A., Cibin, V., Barrucci, F., Pernthaler, J., Corno, G., & Ricci, A. (2018). Assessing the Influence of Vegan, Vegetarian and Omnivore Oriented Westernized Dietary Styles on Human Gut Microbiota: A Cross Sectional Study. *Frontiers in microbiology*, 9, 317. https://doi.org/10.3389/fmicb.2018.00317

11 Sapone, A., Bai, J. C., Ciacci, C., Dolinsek, J., Green, P. H., Hadjivassiliou, M., Kaukinen, K., Rostami, K., Sanders, D. S., Schumann, M., Ullrich, R., Villalta, D., Volta, U., Catassi, C., & Fasano, A. (2012). Spectrum of gluten-related disorders: consensus on new nomenclature and classification. *BMC medicine*, 10, 13. https://doi.org/10.1186/1741-7015-10-13

Chapter 11

1 Neufer, P. D., Costill, D. L., Flynn, M. G., Kirwan, J. P., Mitchell, J. B., & Houmard, J. (1987). Improvements in exercise performance: effects of carbohydrate feedings and diet. *Journal of applied physiology* (Bethesda, Md. : 1985), 62(3), 983–988. https://doi.org/10.1152/jappl.1987.62.3.983

2 Van Proeyen, K., Szlufcik, K., Nielens, H., Ramaekers, M., & Hespel, P. (2011). Beneficial metabolic adaptations due to endurance exercise training in the fasted state. *Journal of applied physiology* (Bethesda, Md. : 1985), 110(1), 236–245. https://doi.org/10.1152/japplphysiol.00907.2010

3 Hawley, J. A., & Burke, L. M. (1997). Effect of meal frequency and timing on physical performance. *The British journal of nutrition*, 77 Suppl 1, S91–S103. https://doi.org/10.1079/bjn19970107

4 Galloway, S. D., Lott, M. J., & Toulouse, L. C. (2014). Preexercise carbohydrate feeding and high-intensity exercise capacity: effects of timing of intake and carbohydrate concentration. *International journal of sport nutrition and exercise metabolism*, 24(3), 258–266. https://doi.org/10.1123/ijsnem.2013-0119

5 Ormsbee, M. J., Bach, C. W., & Baur, D. A. (2014). Pre-exercise nutrition: the role of macronutrients, modified starches and supplements on metabolism and endurance performance. *Nutrients*, 6(5), 1782–1808. https://doi.org/10.3390/nu6051782

6 Kerksick, C. M., Arent, S., Schoenfeld, B. J., Stout, J. R., Campbell, B., Wilborn, C. D., Taylor, L., Kalman, D., Smith-Ryan, A. E., Kreider, R. B., Willoughby, D., Arciero, P. J., VanDusseldorp, T. A., Ormsbee, M. J., Wildman, R., Greenwood, M., Ziegenfuss, T. N., Aragon, A. A., & Antonio, J. (2017). International society of sports nutrition position stand: nutrient timing. *Journal of the International Society of Sports Nutrition*, 14, 33. https://doi.org/10.1186/s12970-017-0189-4

7 Ivy, J. L., Katz, A. L., Cutler, C. L., Sherman, W. M., & Coyle, E. F. (1988). Muscle glycogen synthesis after exercise: effect of time of carbohydrate ingestion. *Journal of applied physiology* (Bethesda, Md. : 1985), 64(4), 1480–1485. https://doi.org/10.1152/jappl.1988.64.4.1480

8 Nieman, D. C., Davis, J. M., Henson, D. A., Walberg-Rankin, J., Shute, M., Dumke, C. L., Utter, A. C., Vinci, D. M., Carson, J. A., Brown, A., Lee, W. J., McAnulty, S. R., & McAnulty, L. S. (2003). Carbohydrate ingestion influences skeletal muscle cytokine mRNA and plasma cytokine levels after a 3-h run. *Journal of applied physiology* (Bethesda, Md. : 1985), 94(5), 1917–1925. https://doi.org/10.1152/japplphysiol.01130.2002

9 Macnaughton, L. S., Wardle, S. L., Witard, O. C., McGlory, C., Hamilton, D. L., Jeromson, S., Lawrence, C. E., Wallis, G. A., & Tipton, K. D. (2016). The response of muscle protein synthesis following whole-body resistance exercise is greater following 40 g than 20 g of ingested whey protein. *Physiological reports*, 4(15), e12893. https://doi.org/10.14814/phy2.12893

10 Elliot, T. A., Cree, M. G., Sanford, A. P., Wolfe, R. R., & Tipton, K. D. (2006). Milk ingestion stimulates net muscle protein synthesis following resistance exercise. *Medicine and science in sports and exercise*, 38(4), 667–674. https://doi.org/10.1249/01.mss.0000210190.64458.25

11 Areta, J. L., Burke, L. M., Ross, M. L., Camera, D. M., West, D. W., Broad, E. M., Jeacocke, N. A., Moore, D. R., Stellingwerff, T., Phillips, S. M., Hawley, J. A., & Coffey, V. G. (2013). Timing and distribution of protein ingestion during prolonged recovery from resistance exercise alters myofibrillar protein synthesis. *The Journal of physiology*, 591(9), 2319–2331. https://doi.org/10.1113/jphysiol.2012.244897

12 Potter, G. D., Skene, D. J., Arendt, J., Cade, J. E., Grant, P. J., & Hardie, L. J. (2016). Circadian Rhythm and Sleep Disruption: Causes, Metabolic Consequences, and Countermeasures. *Endocrine reviews*, 37(6), 584–608. https://doi.org/10.1210/er.2016-1083

13 Stenvers, D. J., Scheer, F., Schrauwen, P., la Fleur, S. E., & Kalsbeek, A. (2019). Circadian clocks and insulin resistance. Nature reviews. *Endocrinology*, 15(2), 75–89. https://doi.org/10.1038/s41574-018-0122-1

14 Pot, G. K., Hardy, R., & Stephen, A. M. (2016). Irregularity of energy intake at meals: prospective associations with the metabolic syndrome in adults of the 1946 British birth cohort. *The British journal of nutrition*, 115(2), 315–323. https://doi.org/10.1017/S0007114515004407

15 Heo, J., Choi, WJ., Ham, S. *et al.* Association between breakfast skipping and metabolic outcomes by sex, age, and work status stratification. *Nutr Metab (Lond)* 18, 8

(2021). https://doi.org/10.1186/s12986-020-00526-z

16 Ofori-Asenso, R., Owen, A. J., & Liew, D. (2019). Skipping Breakfast and the Risk of Cardiovascular Disease and Death: A Systematic Review of Prospective Cohort Studies in Primary Prevention Settings. *Journal of cardiovascular development and disease, 6*(3), 30. https://doi.org/10.3390/jcdd6030030

17 Collado, M. C., Engen, P. A., Bandín, C., Cabrera-Rubio, R., Voigt, R. M., Green, S. J., Naqib, A., Keshavarzian, A., Scheer, F., & Garaulet, M. (2018). Timing of food intake impacts daily rhythms of human salivary microbiota: a randomized, crossover study. *FASEB journal : official publication of the Federation of American Societies for Experimental Biology, 32*(4), 2060–2072. https://doi.org/10.1096/fj.201700697RR

18 Yoshida, J., Eguchi, E., Nagaoka, K., Ito, T., & Ogino, K. (2018). Association of night eating habits with metabolic syndrome and its components: a longitudinal study. *BMC public health, 18*(1), 1366. https://doi.org/10.1186/s12889-018-6262-3

19 Gill, S., & Panda, S. (2015). A Smartphone App Reveals Erratic Diurnal Eating Patterns in Humans that Can Be Modulated for Health Benefits. *Cell metabolism, 22*(5), 789–798. https://doi.org/10.1016/j.cmet.2015.09.005

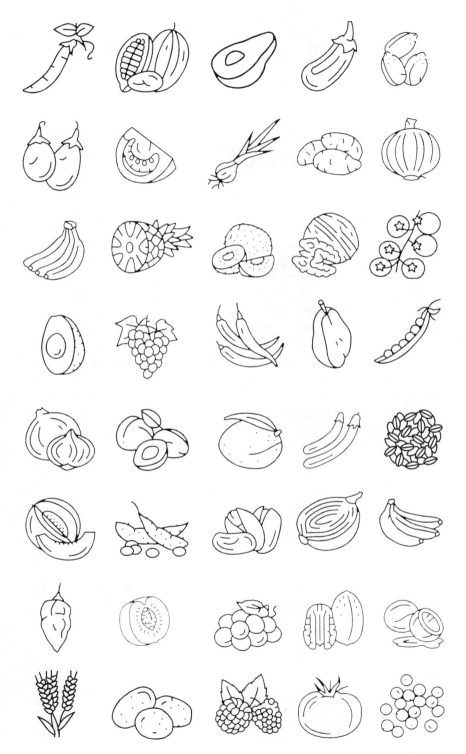

RECIPES

There are so many good vegan recipes available now. I remember, even 10 years ago, how few vegan cookbooks were available and how the vegan option was usually either pasta with tomato sauce or lentils and rice. Now you'll find innovative vegan food all over the internet, social media and in restaurants everywhere. We've come a long way in a short time!

These few recipes are ones that I particularly like myself and cook often. Although there are seven breakfasts, seven lunches and seven dinners, don't think of this as a meal plan for a week, as the calories and macros probably won't be appropriate for your situation. I've included the macro information so that if you want to use the recipe as part of your nutrition plan you can.

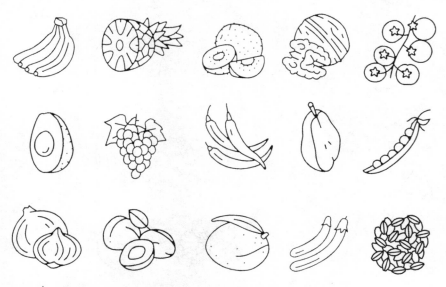

BREAKFAST

APPLE PIE PROTEIN PORRIDGE

Serves 1

Calories per serving - 332
Protein - 29g
Carbs - 41g
Fats - 6g

Ingredients

For the porridge:

- 1 cup (225ml) almond milk (or your favorite plant milk)
- 2/3 cup (50g) steel cut oats
- 1 scoop vegan protein powder
- ½ apple, chopped
- 1 tsp ground cinnamon
- 1 cinnamon stick
- Vanilla extract (optional)

For the toppings:

- Chopped hazelnuts or almonds
- Blueberries
- 1 tbs maple syrup (optional)

Method

Add the oats and cinnamon stick to 200ml of almond milk in a saucepan.

Heat until everything's boiling and then bring it down to a simmer, stirring until you get a thick consistency.

Take the porridge off the heat and remove the cinnamon stick. Once it's cooled a little add the remaining almond milk, protein powder, cinnamon, chopped apples, vanilla extract if using (a couple of drops) and stir well.

Add your toppings, and drizzle over the maple syrup, if you're using it.

BREAKFAST POTATOES

Serves 2

Calories per serving - 423
Protein - 15g
Carbs - 51g
Fats - 19g

Ingredients

- 2 tbsp olive oil
- 3 medium potatoes (approx. 14 oz/400g)
- 2 medium onions
- 7 oz (200g) firm tofu
- 1 tsp ground cumin
- 2 tsp dried oregano
- 1 tsp salt
- 1 tsp black pepper
- ½ cup cherry tomatoes

Method

Cut the potatoes into small cubes. Peel the onions, cut the onions in half, and then slice into half rings.

Heat the oil over a medium heat and cook the potatoes for a few minutes, stirring all the time. Once the potatoes start to sweat, add the onions and cook for a minute or so.

Using your hands, crumble the tofu into the pan, add salt, pepper, cumin and oregano and stir well. Cover and cook for about 15 minutes – you can add more oil or a little hot water if it gets too dry.

Cut the tomatoes in half and fry them over a medium heat in another pan, using a little oil.

Assemble the potatoes and tomatoes on a plate.

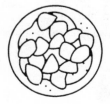

OVERNIGHT OATS WITH PEANUT BUTTER AND BANANA

Serves 1

Calories per serving - 623
Protein - 21g
Carbs - 86g
Fats - 26g

Ingredients

For the overnight oats:

- ¾ cup old-fashioned oats
- ½ banana
- 2 tbsp peanut butter
- 1 tbsp maple syrup
- ½ to ¾ cups plant milk

For the toppings:

- ½ banana, sliced
- 2 tbsp peanut butter

Method

Put the oats in a jar or another large container

Mash half the banana, add peanut butter and maple syrup. Mix well.

Add the milk to the oats, and the banana and peanut butter mixture, and mix well.

Screw the lid on the jar, or seal the container tightly, and refrigerate overnight.

Top with peanut butter and banana slices.

CHICKPEA AVOCADO TOAST

Serve 2

Calories per serving - 507
Protein - 16g
Carbs - 57g
Fats - 26g

Ingredients

- 1 16 oz (400g) can chickpeas
- 1 tbsp extra virgin olive oil and more to drizzle
- 1 tsp turmeric
- 1 avocado
- 2 slices bread (use sourdough or multigrain)
- Sal and pepper
- Squeeze of lemon juice

Method

Drain, rinse and pat the chickpeas dry with kitchen towel.

Heat the olive oil, add the chickpeas and cook over a medium heat for several minutes, stirring continuously. Add the turmeric and stir until the chickpeas are coated.

Cook for a several more minutes until the chickpeas are nicely cooked, then remove from the heat. Add a squeeze of lemon, some salt, and shake.

Mash the avocado with a fork, season with salt and pepper, and spread over the toasted bread. Top it all with the roasted chickpeas and drizzle with extra virgin olive oil.

BREAKFAST QUINOA WITH CHOCOLATE AND PEANUT BUTTER

Serves 1

Calories per serving - 650
Protein - 19g
Carbs - 97g
Fats - 22g

Ingredients

- ½ (90g) cup quinoa
- 1 ½ cups (350ml) soy milk or any plant milk of your choice
- 2 tbsp peanut butter
- 1 ½ tbsp cocoa powder
- 1 ½ tbsp maple syrup, brown rice syrup or sweetener of choice (optional)

Method

Put the quinoa and soy milk in a pan and cook over a medium over medium-low heat. Cover and cook for 15-20 minutes, until quinoa is cooked through, stirring occasionally.

Remove from the heat and stir in the peanut butter, cocoa powder and maple syrup.

SCRAMBLED TOFU BREAKFAST BURRITO

Serves 4

Calories per serving - 441
Protein - 16.5g
Carbs - 53.5g
Fats - 19.5g

Ingredients

- 12oz (340g) firm or extra-firm tofu
- 5 (750g) whole baby potatoes, chopped
- 1 medium red bell pepper, thinly sliced
- 2 cups (134g) kale, chopped
- 2 tsp oil (or 2 tbsp (30 ml) water)
- 3 cloves (9 g) garlic, minced
- 1 tbsp (15g) hummus
- 1 tsp chili powder
- 1 tsp cumin
- 1 tsp nutritional yeast
- Sea salt
- 1 pinch cayenne pepper (optional)
- ¼ cup (15g) minced parsley
- 3-4 large whole wheat tortillas
- 1 medium avocado, mashed
- Cilantro
- Salsa or hot sauce

Method

Preheat oven to 400 degrees F (200 C).

Put the potatoes and peppers on a baking sheet (lined with parchment paper), drizzle with oil (or water), ½ tsp cumin, ½ tsp chili powder, salt and toss together to combine. Bake for 15-20 minutes.

Wrap the tofu in a clean dishtowel and press it with something heavy to remove the excess moisture. Crumble it into fine pieces with a fork.

In the last 5 minutes of baking the potatoes and peppers, add the kale so that wilts, and combine it with the other vegetables and spices.

Sauté the tofu with garlic in a pan over a medium heat, using either the oil or water, for 8-10 minutes.

While it's cooking, combine hummus, ½ tsp chili powder, ½ tsp cumin, nutritional yeast, ¼ tsp salt and cayenne pepper if you're using it in a small bowl. Add water in small amounts (up to about 3 tbsp) until the sauce is pourable, and the add parsley and mix well. Add this to the tofu and continue cooking over a medium heat for 3-5 minutes.

To assemble the burritos, add the roasted vegetables, tofu, mashed avocado, cilantro and salsa to a large wholewheat tortilla, and roll up!

FLUFFY VEGAN PROTEIN PANCAKES

Serves 2

Calories per serving - 295
Protein - 16g
Carbs - 60g
Fats - 1,.2g

Ingredients

For the pancakes:

- 1 cup (120 g) all-purpose flour
- 1/4 cup (28 g) vegan protein powder of choice
- 1 tbsp baking powder
- 1/2 tsp sea salt
- 2 tbsp maple syrup (optional)
- 1 cup water

For the toppings:

- Sliced banana
- Blueberries

Method

Combine flour, protein powder, baking powder and salt in a bowl.

If you're using it add the maple syrup, and slowly add water, until it is just mixed – it shouldn't be too smooth and runny, but thick and pourable. You can use more than 1 cup of water if needed. Let the batter rest (5-10 minutes).

Heat a pan over a medium to low heat. Either use a non-stick pan, or a little oil or cooking spray, and use about ¼ of the batter for each pancake.

When bubbles start to form and the edges of the pancakes are starting to cook through, flip the pancakes and cook for another couple of minutes.

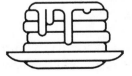

LUNCH

TEMPEH SANDWICH

Serves 2

Calories per serving - 547
Protein - 21g
Carbs - 51g
Fats - 32g

Ingredients

- 4 slices wholegrain bread
- 3 oz (80g) tempeh
- 2 handfuls arugula (rocket)
- ½ cup (100g) sun-dried tomatoes in oil
- 1 tbsp olive oil
- 2 tbsp vinegar (balsamic, malt or wine vinegar)
- 2 tbsp soy sauce
- 2 tsp maple syrup
- 1 avocado
- Juice of half a lemon
- Salt and pepper

Method

Slice the tempeh into 8 slices. Fry in oil for a couple of minutes, then add the soy sauce, vinegar and maple syrup.

Turn the tempeh, making sure it is covered in the sauces and cook for a few more minutes.

Mash the avocado in a bowl with the lemon juice, salt and pepper, then spread it over 2 slices of bread.

Assemble the sandwiches by placing rocket, chopped sun dried tomatoes and tempeh on the other slices of bread. Top with the avocado bread.

PEANUT CRUNCH SALAD

Serves 4

Calories per serving - 376
Protein - 20g
Carbs - 44g
Fats - 23g

Ingredients

For the quinoa:

- 1 cup (180g) quinoa (2 cups (370g) already cooked quinoa)
- 1¾ cup (420 ml) water
- salt

For the dressing:

- 5 tbsp peanut butter
- 4 tbsp lemon juice
- 2 tbsp soy sauce
- 4 tbsp water
- 2 tbsp vinegar (rice wine or apple cider/white wine vinegar)
- 1-2 tbsp maple syrup (optional)
- salt and pepper

For the salad:

- 4 green onions (spring onions)
- 1 medium carrot
- 1 cup (150g) edamame beans
- 1½ cups (160g) red cabbage
- 1½ cups (160g) green cabbage
- ½ cup (73g) roasted peanuts (salted or unsalted)

Method

Boil the water and add the quinoa with a pinch of salt. Cover it and turn the heat right down and cook for 15 minutes. Turn it off and let it stand for 10 minutes without removing the lid.

Make the dressing by adding all the dressing ingredients together and mixing well.

Slice the green onions into thin rounds, cut the carrot into matchsticks (or grate it), chop the red and the green cabbage and combine with all the rest of the ingredients, the edamame, quinoa and dressing.

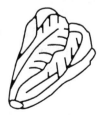

VEGAN PASTA ARRABIATA

Serves 2

Calories per serving - 421
Protein - 15g
Carbs - 70g
Fats - 14g

Ingredients

- 1 small aubergine
- ¼ tsp salt
- 8 oz (250g) whole wheat pasta
- ¼ tsp paprika
- 1 medium onion
- 2 cloves garlic, minced
- 2 medium tomatoes
- ¼ tsp sugar
- 1 tbsp olive oil
- 1 tsp tomato paste
- 2 cups (500ml) tomato juice
- 1 red chili pepper
- 2 tbsp almonds (roasted or smoked), chopped

Method

Cook the pasta according to the instructions on the package.

Cut the aubergine into small evenly sized pieces and cook over a medium heat with a little olive oil, adding salt and paprika, stir for a couple of minutes.

Dice the onion and add to the aubergine and fry until the onion softens. Add the minced garlic and fry for a few moments, then add the tomato paste and cook for a few more minutes.

Add the tomato juice, the tomato pieces, the sugar and the chili pepper, finely chopped, and cook for another fix minutes, stirring.

Serve the sauce over the pasta and garnish with almonds.

SWEET POTATO TOFU BOWLS

Serves 4

Calories per serving - 583
Protein - 26g
Carbs - 49g
Fats - 34g

Ingredients

- For the Pickled Red Onion:
- 1 red onion, thinly sliced
- ½ cup (118 ml) white vinegar
- ½ cup (118 ml) water
- 1 tbsp sugar
- ½ tsp sea salt

For the Mint Cilantro Dressing:

- ½ cup (80g) hemp seeds
- ½ (118 ml) cup water
- ¼ cup (4g) picked cilantro leaves
- ¼ cup (4g) picked mint leaves

- 2 tbsp lime juice
- 2 cloves garlic
- 1 tbsp olive oil
- ½ tsp salt
- Pepper

For the Sweet Potato Tofu Bowls:

- 350g extra firm tofu, cubed
- 2 tbsp soy sauce or tamari
- 1 tsp cayenne
- 1 tsp garlic powder
- 2 cups (260g) sweet potato, chopped into cubes
- 4 tsp olive oil
- 1 tsp chilli flakes
- salt and pepper
- 1 tsp smoked paprika
- 4 cups (270g) kale
- 2 tbsp lemon juice
- 1 cup (185g) cooked quinoa
- 1 cup (200g) cooked green lentils
- 2 avocados

Method

To make the pickled red onion, boil water and pour into a container large enough for the red onion. Add vinegar, salt and sugar and stir well, the add the red onion, making sure that it's covered by the water. Leave for 30 minutes at least.

Cook the lentils and quinoa according to the instructions on the packages. Preheat the oven to 375°F (190°C)

Mix the tofu, cayenne, garlic powder, soy sauce, salt and pepper in a bowl, to coat the tofu and then spread it out evenly over a lined baking tray. Bake for 20-25 minutes.

Mix the cubed sweet potato with 2 tsp of the olive oil, chili flakes, smoked paprika and some salt and pepper so that the sweet potato is thoroughly coated. Spread the sweet potato out evenly over a baking tray and bake for 20-30 minutes.

To make the dressing, use a blender to blend all the ingredients listed until it's a smooth consistency. If you're not using it immediately, store in an airtight container.

Chop the kale and put it into a bowl with 2 tsp of olive oil and 2 tbsp of lemon juice and massage with your hands until it is softened.

Divide the kale, lentils, quinoa, sweet potato and tofu between 4 bowls, top with sliced avocado, pickled red onions and dressing when you're ready to eat!

FARRO PROTEIN BOWL

Serves 2

Calories per serving - 423
Protein - 21g
Carbs - 69g
Fats - 15g

Ingredients

- 1 cup (133g) diced sweet potatoes
- 1 cup (150g) diced carrots
- 2 tsp olive oil
- 15 oz (400g) can chickpeas, drained and rinsed
- 4 oz (100g) smoky tempeh strips
- 2 ½ (590ml) cups water
- 1 cup (240g) uncooked farro
- Salt & pepper
- 2 cups (150g) mixed greens
- ½ cup (125g) hummus
- ¼ cup (40g) roasted almonds
- 2 lemon wedges

Method

Preheat the oven to 375°F (190°C).

Mix the sweet potatoes and carrots with 1 tsp olive oil, and some salt & pepper. Spread them out evenly on one third of a large baking sheet.

Mix the chickpeas with 1 tsp olive oil and some salt & pepper.

Spread out evenly on the middle third of the same baking sheet as the sweet potatoes and carrots.

Place the tempeh strips on the remaining third of the baking sheet. Roast everything in the oven for 30 minutes, turning the tempeh halfway through and stirring the sweet potato and chickpeas without letting them mix together.

Put the farro and 2 ½ cups of water (with a pinch of salt) into a pan and bring to the boil. Cover and reduce to a medium-low heat. Cook for 20-25 minutes – it should be soft but still chewy.

Once everything is cooked, divide it all between 2 bowls, adding the greens, and top with hummus and almonds. Squeeze over the lemon from the wedges when you're ready to eat!

CREAMY SWEET CORN PAPPARDELLE

Serves 4

Calories per serving - 603
Protein - 20g
Carbs - 97g
Fats - 18g

Ingredients

- 2 tbsp extra-virgin olive oil
- ½ cup (26g) chopped yellow onion
- 4 cups (650g) sweetcorn
- 2 garlic cloves, crushed
- ½ (70g) cup raw cashews
- ¼ cup (60ml) water
- 2 tbsp lemon juice
- ¼ tsp smoked paprika
- ½ tsp sea salt
- Black pepper
- 12 oz (340g) pappardelle or pasta of choice
- 2 green onions, finely sliced
- 3 packed cups fresh spinach
- ½ cup sliced fresh basil, for serving (optional)

Method

Heat 1 tbsp of oil in pan over a medium heat and cook the onion for a few minutes until soft. Add garlic, and 1 ½ cups of corn and cook for a few more minutes. If you're using corn from the cob, cook until tender.

Put the cooked corn and onion into a blender and add cashews, water, lemon juice, paprika, ½ salt and some pepper. Blend until smooth, scraping down the sides and adding more water if necessary.

Cook the pasta according to the instructions on the package. Drain the pasta but keep aside ½ cup of pasta water.

Heat 1 tbsp of oil in a pan over a medium heat, add the green onions and the rest of the corn (and some salt and pepper). Cook until everything softens, then add the spinach, cooked pasta, blended corn and enough of the reserved pasta water to make a creamy sauce.

Serve with sliced basil to garnish.

VEGAN "MEATBALL" SUB

Serves 4

Calories per serving - 498
Protein - 29g
Carbs - 66g
Fats - 11g

Ingredients

- 14 oz (400g) vegan mince
- 2 garlic cloves, minced
- Parsley
- Salt & pepper
- 18 0z (500g) passata
- 4 sub rolls (wholegrain if possible)
- 4½ oz (120g) vegan mozzarella, grated
- Fresh basil

Method

Mix vegan mince with garlic, parsley, salt and pepper and combine thoroughly. Using your hands, make the "meatballs" about the size of a golf ball.

Fry the meatballs in some oil, turning regularly until they are nicely browned all over (about 10 minutes)

Add the passata to the pan, stir the meatballs in and allow to simmer for 5-10 minutes, so that the sauce can thicken.

Cut the subs lengthways to make room for the meatballs, and when everything is cooked, place the meatballs in a row, adding sauce to each one.

Sprinkle the grated vegan mozzarella over the meatballs and put the subs under a grill for a couple of minutes to melt the cheese.

Serve with basil to garnish.

DINNER

SWEET POTATO & CAULIFLOWER LENTIL BOWL

Serves 4

Calories per serving - 350
Protein - 15g
Carbs - 41g
Fats - 11g

Ingredients

- 1 large sweet potato
- 1 cauliflower
- 1 tbsp garam masala
- 3 tbsp olive oil
- 2 cloves garlic
- 7 oz (200g) puy lentils
- 2-inch piece of ginger, grated
- 1 tsp mustard (Dijon)
- Pinch of sugar
- 1½ limes, juiced
- 2 carrots
- ¼ red cabbage
- 1 oz (30g) cilantro

Method

Preheat oven to 400°F (200°C).

Cut the sweet potato into medium chunks and the cauliflower into large florets, dicing the stalk. Toss with the garlic, garam masala and 1½ tbsp of olive oil, and spread evenly over a large baking sheet. Roast for 30-35 minutes.

Bring the lentils to boil in 400ml water and simmer for 20-25 minutes until the lentils cooked through, but completely soft, then drain.

Take the garlic cloves from the roasted vegetables, crush with the blade of a knife and out it into a bowl with 1½ tbsp of olive oil, grated ginger, mustard, sugar, juice of ½ lime. Stir until thoroughly combined.

Add the dressing to the warm lentils and stir, adding salt and pepper to taste. Grate the carrots, shred the red cabbage and chop the cilantro, squeeze over the juice of 1 lime, and mix well, also adding salt and pepper to taste.

To serve, divide everything between 4 bowls, lentils underneath the sweet potato and cauliflower, topping with the carrots and cabbage.

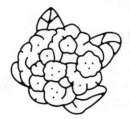

GRILLED TOFU, BROCCOLI, AND RICE BOWL

Serves 4

Calories per serving - 470
Protein - 29g
Carbs - 55g
Fats - 17g

Ingredients

- 24 oz (680g) firm tofu
- 16 oz (450g) brown rice
- 4 cups (10oz/280g) broccoli
- 1 can (15 oz/400g) black beans, drained and rinsed
- 4 tbsp nutritional yeast
- ½ tsp black pepper
- ½ tsp salt
- 2 tbsp olive oil

Method

Cut the tofu into even slices and pat dry. Sprinkle with 2 tbsp nutritional yeast and ¼ tsp black pepper.

Heat a grill pan to medium heat and add a little oil or cooking spray and grill the tofu for several minutes on each side, until it starts to get crispy.

Meanwhile, steam the broccoli until tender.

Mix the rice and drained beans with 2 tbsp olive oil, 2 tbsp nutritional yeast, ¼ tsp black pepper, and salt.

Divide the rice and beans between 4 bowls, add the broccoli and top with tofu.

Portion out your rice mixture onto four plates or meal prep containers and top each with 3 pieces of grilled tofu.

CURRY RED LENTIL STEW WITH KALE & CHICKPEAS

Serves 6

Calories per serving - 355
Protein - 21.5g
Carbs - 60g
Fats - 5g

Ingredients

- 1 tbsp olive oil (or 1/4 cup water/veg broth)
- 1 large yellow onion, diced
- 5 cloves garlic, minced
- 1 ½ inch fresh ginger, minced
- 1–2 tbsp curry powder (to taste)
- 1 tsp cumin
- 1 tsp turmeric
- salt
- 1-2 tsp red pepper flakes (optional)
- 1 can (15 oz/400g) fire roasted tomatoes or 1 cup fresh tomatoes, diced
- 2 cups (380g) dry red lentils,

rinsed and picked over

- 1 can (15 oz/400g) garbanzo beans, drained and rinsed
- 6 cups (1.4 liters) water or vegetable broth, + more as needed
- 4 cups (260g) kale, julienned
- 1 lemon, juiced (optional)

To serve:

- Brown rice (or basmati)

Method

Heat 1 tbsp olive oil in a large pot over a medium heat. Add onion, garlic and ginger and sauté until the onion is soft and transparent.

Add the curry powder, cumin and turmeric and stir with the onions briefly. Then add the tomatoes, lentils, garbanzo beans and 6 cups of the vegetable broth. Bring everything to the boil, cover and simmer for 30 minutes.

Add the kale and the lemon juice (if using) and cook until the kale softens (about 10 minutes).

Serve over rice.

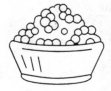

VEGAN CHILLI

Serves 6

Calories per serving - 412
Protein - 27g
Carbs - 37g
Fats - 17g

Ingredients

- 2 tbsp olive oil
- 3 cloves garlic, minced
- 1 large red onion, thinly sliced
- 2 celery stalks, finely chopped
- 2 medium carrots, peeled and finely chopped
- 2 red peppers, roughly chopped
- 1 tsp ground cumin
- 1 tsp chili powder
- Salt and pepper
- 2 cans (30 oz/800g) chopped tomatoes
- 1 can (15 oz/400g) red kidney beans, drained and rinsed
- 3.5 oz (100g) split red lentils
- 14 oz (400g) soy mince (frozen works)
- 1 cup (250 ml) vegetable stock
- 1 tsp miso paste (optional)
- 2 tbsp balsamic vinegar (optional)
- A large handful of fresh cilantro, roughly chopped (optional)

To serve

- Brown rice (or basmati)
- Chopped cilantro
- Squeeze of lime juice

Method

Heat 2 tbsp olive oil in a large pot over a medium heat. Add the onion, garlic, celery, carrots and peppers and sauté for a couple of minutes.

Add cumin, chili powder, salt and pepper and stir briefly. Then add the 2 cans of chopped tomatoes, kidney beans, lentils, soy mince and 1 cup vegetable stock. Add the miso, balsamic vinegar and chopped cilantro, if using.

Bring to a boil, then cover and simmer for 25 minutes.

Serve over rice, sprinkled with cilantro and a squeeze of lime.

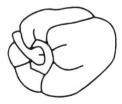

HIGH PROTEIN PESTO PASTA RECIPE

Serves 4

Calories per serving - 420
Protein - 20g
Carbs - 49g
Fats - 18g

Ingredients

- 8 oz (227g) high protein chickpea or lentil pasta
- 1 can (14oz/400g) artichoke hearts, drained
- 4 cups (120g) baby spinach
- ½ cup (27g) sundried tomatoes, (packed in oil & drained)

For the spirulina pesto:

- 2 tbsp spirulina powder
- ¼ cup (33g) raw sunflower seeds
- 1 cup (20g) packed basil leaves
- 1 cup (25g) packed parsley leaves, stems on
- 1/3 cup (80ml) olive oil (or avocado oil)
- 2 cloves garlic
- 2 tbsp apple cider vinegar
- 6 tbsp lemon juice + zest
- Salt and pepper

To serve:

- Sunflower seeds, toasted
- Vegan parmesan, grated

Method

Prepare the pasta according to the instructions on the package, once it's cooked, drain but reserve about ¼-½ cup of the pasta water.

Add all the ingredients for the spirulina pesto to a food processor. Blend until to the consistency of a pesto, adding more liquid (lemon juice or apple cider vinegar) if needed.

Roughly chop the artichokes and sundried tomatoes, add them to a pan over a medium heat and cook for a couple of minutes. Add the spinach and cook until it is just wilted, then add the cooked pasta, the pesto and a little pasta water – adding more as needed so that it mixes well.

Garnish with toasted sunflower seeds and your choice of grated vegan cheese.

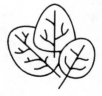

VEGAN FIESTA TACO BOWL

Serves 4

Calories per serving - 744
Protein - 28g
Carbs - 50g
Fats - 52g

Ingredients

For the dressing:

- ½ cup (17g) chopped fresh cilantro
- ⅓ cup (80ml) extra-virgin olive oil
- ¼ cup (60ml) lime juice
- 2 tbsp agave nectar (or sweetener of choice)
- 1 jalapeño, seeded
- ¼ tsp sea salt
- ¼ tsp freshly ground black pepper

For the lime "sour cream":

- 1 cup silken tofu
- ¼ cup (60ml) extra-virgin olive oil
- 2 tbsp lime juice
- ½ tsp sea salt

For the taco bowls:

- 2 tbsp extra-virgin olive oil
- 8 oz (227g) ground seitan
- 1 tsp chili powder
- 1 tsp smoked paprika
- Pinch of cayenne pepper

- Salt
- 2 heads (about 15 oz/425g) romaine lettuce, cut or torn into bite-size pieces
- 1 cup (6.5oz/185g) cooked quinoa (made from about 1/3 cup or 60g uncooked quinoa)
- 1 cup (6oz/172g) cooked black beans, (from a can, drained and rinsed)
- 1 cup (6oz/170g) sweet corn
- 1 cup (5oz/140g) halved cherry tomatoes
- 1 avocado, mashed

To serve:

- Crispy tortilla strips
- Lime wedges

Method

To make the dressing, combine all the ingredients in a food processor and blend until smooth. You make the lime "sour cream" the same way – place all the ingredients in a food processor and blend until smooth. Store both in separate airtight containers.

Heat 2 tbsp olive oil in a large pan over a medium heat, cook the seitan, chili powder, smoked paprika and cayenne and cook through. Add a little water if it starts to look dry.

Combine romaine lettuce, black beans, sweetcorn, tomatoes and quinoa in a bowl and mix with the dressing until everything is coated. Divide into 4 bowls, and top with seitan, mashed avocado, lime "sour cream" and tortilla strips. Garnish with extra lime wedges.

VEGAN BUTTERNUT MAC AND "CHEESE" WITH SMOKY SHIITAKE "BACON"

Serves 6

Calories per serving - 717
Protein - 21g
Carbs - 110g
Fats - 23g

Ingredients

For the smoky shiitake "bacon":

- 1 cup (4oz/113g) shiitake mushrooms, stemmed and thinly sliced
- 2 tbsp extra-virgin olive oil
- ¼ tsp salt
- ¼ tsp smoked paprika
- ¼ tsp garlic powder

For the mac and "cheese":

- 5 cups (20oz/567g) peeled and cubed butternut squash
- 2 tbsp extra-virgin olive oil
- 2 cups water

- Black pepper
- 2¼ tsp sea salt, divided
- 1 pound (454g) elbow macaroni
- ½ cup (2.5oz/70g) raw cashews
- 1 clove garlic
- ½ tsp dried rosemary
- Smoked paprika, for serving

Method

Preheat the oven to 375°F (190°C).

Mix the mushrooms with olive oil and salt and arrange in a single layer on a lined baking sheet and bake, turning several times, until very crispy (20-30 minutes). When they're cooked, sprinkle with smoked paprika and garlic powder, mix well and set aside.

Turn the oven up to 400°F (200°C). Combine butternut squash with 2 tbsp of olive oil, ¼ tsp salt and pepper, spread on a baking tray and roast for 30 minutes or until tender. Turn occasionally while cooking.

Cook the macaroni in salted boiling water until it is al dente. Drain, retaining ½ cup of the pasta water, and return to the pot.

Add the butternut squash, 2 cups water, cashews, garlic, rosemary and 2 tsp salt to a food processor and blend until smooth. Pour into the pot containing the pasta and mix until combined, adding more of the pasta water if it needs more liquid. Taste and season if necessary.

Garnish with smoky shiitake "bacon" and a sprinkle of smoked paprika.

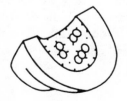

SNACKS

BREAKFAST PROTEIN BARS

Makes 12

Calories per serving - 340
Protein - 10g
Carbs - 21g
Fats - 27g

Ingredients

- 1 cup (3.35oz/95g) desiccated coconut
- ½ cup (2oz/60g) hulled hemp seeds
- ½ cup (2.5oz/70g) sesame seeds
- ½ cup (2oz/60g) pumpkin seeds
- 1 ½ cups (8oz/225g) mixed nuts, chopped into small chunks (eg. cashews, walnuts, almonds, pecans, pistachios)
- ½ cup (2.8oz/80g) raisins
- 1 tsp ground cinnamon
- ½ cup (4.5oz/125g) cashew butter, or nut butter of your choice
- 4 tbsp sweetener (maple syrup, date paste etc)
- 1 tsp vanilla extract

Method

Preheat the oven to 350°F (180°C)

Combine desiccated coconut, all the seeds, nuts, raisins and cinnamon in a large bowl.

Heat cashew butter and maple syrup in a pan over a medium heat and stir until it is smooth. Take it off the heat, add vanilla extract and stir well.

Add the cashew mix to the bowl and mix until combined, adding a little water if needed for consistency.

Put in a brownie tin that has been lined with parchment paper and press down evenly into a flat layer.

Bake for 15 minutes, or until golden.

Once cool, cut into 12 bars.

PEANUT BUTTER BLISS BALLS

Makes 12

Calories per serving - 121
Protein - 7g
Carbs - 11g
Fats - 6g

Ingredients

- 1 ½ cups (8oz/225g) dates, pitted
- 7oz (200g) white beans, cooked & drained
- 4 oz (113g) peanut butter
- 2oz (57g) oats
- 2oz (57g) vegan protein powder
- 4 tbsp cocoa powder
- Salt

Optional add-ins

- Roasted peanuts
- Chocolate chips
- Cinnamon
- Vanilla extract

Method

If the dates are not soft, soak them in a bowl of hot water for 15 minutes.

Combine white beans and dates in a food processor and blend for a couple of minutes.

Add the rest of the ingredients and blend until everything is well combined, scraping down the sides as needed.

If it's too sticky, add a little more oats to make a mouldable dough.

With wet hands roll the dough into bite-sized balls. Put in the fridge so that the balls firm up.

VEGAN PROTEIN CHIA PUDDING

3 servings

Calories per serving - 259
Protein - 8g
Carbs - 30g
Fats - 13g

Ingredients

- 6 tbsp chia seeds
- 2½ cups (590ml) plant milk
- 2 scoops vanilla vegan protein powder (if you use chocolate subtract 2 tbsp cacao powder)
- 6 tbsp cacao powder
- 2 tbsp sweetener (maple syrup, date paste etc, optional)

Optional toppings

- Chocolate chips
- Chopped banana/ strawberry/mango
- Shredded coconut

Method

Add all the ingredients to a food processor. Blend until smooth

If the protein powder is unsweetened, add some sweetener.

Divide between 3 containers and put in the fridge for at least 30 minutes.

Top with some of the optional add-ons.

SPICY & CRUNCHY ROASTED CHICKPEAS

4 servings

Calories per serving - 248
Protein - 11g
Carbs - 37g
Fats - 7g

Ingredients

- 1 can (14oz/400g) cooked chickpeas
- 1 tbsp extra virgin olive oil
- ½ tsp garlic powder
- ½ tsp rosemary
- ¼ tsp cayenne pepper
- ¼ tsp salt

Method

Drain and rinse the chickpeas.

Remove excess water by patting with kitchen towels and leave to dry for an hour.

Pre-heat the oven to 400°F (200°C)

Combine chickpeas with the olive oil, spread evenly on a baking tray.

Roast for 45 minutes or until golden and crispy and remove from the oven.

Mix all the spices, toss with the chickpeas, and shake well.

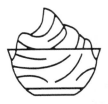